W0050707

Agents and Actions Supplements
Vol. 49

Series Editor
M.J. Parnham, Bonn

Therapeutic Strategies for Modulating the Inflammatory Diseases

Edited by

B.M. Weichman
A.J. Main
L. Marshall
J. Winkler
L.G. Letts

Springer Basel AG

Editors:

Dr. B.M. Weichman
BMW Associates
86 Richmond Drive
Skillman, NJ 08558
USA

Dr. L. Marshall
Dr. J. Winkler
SmithKline Beecham
709 Swedeland Road
King of Prussia, PA 19406
USA

Dr. A.J. Main
Ciba-Geigy Corporation
556 Morris Avenue
Summit, NJ 07901
USA

Dr. L.G. Letts
NitroMed, Inc.
801 Albany Street
Boston, MA 02118
USA

A CIP catalogue record for this book is available from the Library of Congress,
Washington D.C., USA

Deutsche Bibliothek Cataloging-in-Publication Data

Therapeutic strategies for modulating the inflammatory diseases / ed. by B. M.
Weichman ... – Basel ; Boston ; Berlin : Birkhäuser, 1997
  (Agents and actions : Supplements ; 49)
   ISBN 978-3-0348-9804-1   ISBN 978-3-0348-8857-8 (eBook)
   DOI 10.1007/978-3-0348-8857-8

The publisher and editors can give no guarantee for the information on drug dosage and administration contained in this
publication. The respective user must check its accuracy by consulting other sources of reference in each individual case.

The use of registered names, trademarks, etc. in this publication, even if not identified as such, does not imply that they are
exempt from the relevant protective laws and regulations or free for general use.

This work is subject to copyright. All rights are reserved, whether the whole or part of the material is concerned,
specifically the rights of translation, reprinting, re-use of illustrations, recitation, broadcasting, reproduction on microfilms
or in other ways, and storage in data banks. For any kind of use the permission of the copyright owner must be obtained.

© 1998 Springer Basel AG
Originally published by Birkhäuser Verlag Basel Switzerland in 1998
Softcover reprint of the hardcover 1st edition 1998
Printed on acid-free paper produced from chlorine-free pulp. TCF ∞

ISBN 978-3-0348-9804-1

987654321

Contents

VI

Summaries of workshops and poster discussions

Preface

The Eighth International Conference of the Inflammation Research Association was held on October 27 to 31, 1996 at Hershey Lodge and Convention Center in Hershey, Pennsylvania. As have others in this series, the conference focused on understanding the molecular mechanisms involved in acute and chronic inflammatory reactions as well as on therapeutic approaches to treating inflammatory diseases. One outstanding symposium focused on new drugs and was designed as a forum for the dissemination of early clinical results on new anti-inflammatory agents. Other symposia spotlighted exciting advances being made in defining intracellular signaling pathways and the potential for future therapeutics that target cytokines and costimulatory pathways.

This conference was characterized by a high level of participation by attendees, who represent both the academic and industrial sectors. It was gratifying to note that a large proportion of the attending scientists presented their latest findings during workshops, poster discussions, and poster sessions. This volume covers many of the highlights of the Eighth International Conference and should become a valuable resource for scientists involved in inflammation research and drug discovery.

Barry M. Weichman
Alan J. Main
Lisa Marshall
James Winkler
L. Gordon Letts   August, 1997

AAS 49
Therapeutic Strategies for Modulating the Inflammatory Diseases
© 1998 Birkhäuser Verlag Basel/Switzerland

Targets in cytokine activation

D.A. Giegel[1] and D.D. Chaplin[2]

[1]*Department of Biochemistry, Parke-Davis Research Division, Warner-Lambert Company, Ann Arbor, Michigan, USA*
[2]*Howard Hughes Medical Institute and Washington University School of Medicine, St. Louis, Missouri, USA*

Summary. The first morning session of the Eighth International Conference of the Inflammation Research Association was titled 'Targets in Cytokine Activation'. It encompassed four areas of research that may be considered as either current or future targets. Probably the best established target of the four is interleukin-1β converting enzyme (ICE) and Winnie Wong from BASF Bioresearch Corporation presented an overview of work in this field. This was followed by a newly emerging target called TACE (TNF-α converting enzyme) in a presentation from Douglas Cerretti of Immunex. The final two presentations covered work with chemoattractant receptors (Craig Gerard, Harvard) and mice where the inducible NO synthase gene had been deleted (John Mudgett, Merck).

Perhaps a more appropriate name for the first session of the Eighth International Conference of the Inflammation Research Association would have been 'Targets in Proinflammatory Mediator Activation'. The four mediator systems that were discussed are all thought to occupy positions near the top of the inflammatory cascade. They are either relatively recent targets for antiinflammatory drug discovery or are candidates to be the next generation of targets.

Cloning of interleukin-1β converting enzyme (ICE) was first described in 1992 by groups at both Merck and Immunex. At that time, ICE represented the first example of a mammalian cysteine protease that cleaved after aspartic acid residues (Aspases). ICE is now recognized to define a protease family. In the past four years, there has been an explosive growth of this family which currently numbers ten members that have been isolated from human tissues or cell lines. The family has been given the generic name Caspase by a group of scientists in the field that have been involved in cloning and characterizing the family members. The particular family member is then followed by a number (based on when it was discovered). For example, Caspase-1 is ICE, Caspase-2 is ICH-1 and so on. Dr. Winnie Wong (BASF Bioresearch) reviewed the ICE field, with primary emphasis on the role of these enzymes in regulation of inflammation and with a secondary emphasis on the potentional role of the family members as mediators of apoptosis.

The three-dimensional structures of two of the family members have been solved (CPP32 and ICE) and show striking similarities. Both are tetramers with $(\alpha\beta)_2$ stoichiometry that contain the substrate binding site in grooves along the surface of the enzyme. The main difference between these two enzymes lies out at the P4 position, where CPP32 is more constricted than is ICE. In general, all of the family members contain the sequence QACXG around the active site cysteine and SHG around the catalytic histidine.

Mice that lack the gene for ICE have been generated by gene-targeting. The mice are viable and fertile with no gross abnormalities apparent at any time during their lives. As expected, their monocytes release greatly reduced levels of IL-1β in response to challenge by LPS and ATP. Unexpectedly, they also manifest reduced production of IL-1α. *Ex vivo* experiments with macrophages from these mice suggest that the defect in IL-1α production is mediated by ICE indirectly through a calpain-like protease. ICE-deficient mice also survive a challenge by a dose of LPS that is lethal to wild-type mice. In an acute model of anoxic CNS injury, ICE-deficient mice were found to have a statistically reduced level of brain tissue destruction as compared to wild-type mice.

There now appears to be a cascade of ICE proteases involved in apoptosis. Recently, a new ICE family member was described that contained a protein-protein interaction domain termed a 'death domain'. Caspase-8 or FLICE was found to be involved in Fas-mediated apoptosis by interaction of Caspase-8 and the cytoplasmic domain of Fas *via* this death domain. Ligation of Fas initiated a series of steps that are perphaps reminiscent of the coagulation cascade, whereby Caspase-8 may activate a family member that is similar to ICE in specificity, followed by Mch-2 or Mch-3 and finally activation of CPP32. CPP32 then is thought to deliver the knockout blow to the cell. One of the potential substrates for CPP32 or a related enzyme is thought to be PKC-δ. When this enzyme is cleaved at a Caspase target site, it becomes constitutively active. This catalytic fragment confers a phenotype on HeLa cells that morphologically resembles apoptosis.

The second potential drug target discussed in this session was the TNF-α converting enzyme, or TACE. TNF-α is synthesized as a type II membrane protein. TACE is a metalloprotease that is responsible for the release of TNF-α at the authentic natural cleavage site. TACE was classified as a metalloprotease based on its inhibition by chelators such as EDTA, but it did not fall into the matrix metalloprotease family since it was resistant to inhibition by TIMP-1. A small, synthetic inhibitor of TACE, called TAPI, was developed and shown to prevent lethality in mice treated with LPS plus D-galactosamine.

Attempts to engineer TACE knockout mice showed that this gene deletion is embryonically lethal. For the very few TACE-deficient animals that survive to birth, death occurs within a few weeks. The recognition that mice lacking both the type I and type II TNF receptors are viable suggest that there is another substrate for TACE besides membrane TNF, and that this substrate is crucial to normal embryonic development. Although TACE-deficient animals are nonviable, studies using TACE-deficient cells have shown that they are unable to support release of soluble TNF-α. This supports TACE as the major cellular protease that mediates TNF-α release and suggests that specific TACE inhibitors may be potent systemic blockers of the release of soluble TNF-α.

The chemokine receptors have been long thought of as targets to prevent influx of inflammatory cells at sites of injury. This area of research has recently grown in importance with the realization that the specific chemokine receptor CCR5 is a co-receptor for entry of HIV into the cell. Craig Gerard (Harvard Medical School) began by describing work done in mice carrying a targeted null mutation in the C5a receptor gene. The C5aR -/- mice were viable and appeared grossly normal. They have been studied in a model of acute lung injury. After introduction of a controlled inoculum of live *Pseudomonas* intratracheally, 7/7 wild-type mice survived while 10/11 C5aR-deficient mice died. The high mortality in the C5aR knockout mice appeared to be due to the inability of this mouse strain to clear the bacteria. In the lung, thus, it was found that the C5aR serves non-redundant functions. This is not the case in the skin, where there are several chemo-attractant receptors with overlapping functions. In contrast, mice in which the IL-8R has been deleted show a normal response to *Pseudomonas* challenge.

The chemokine receptor CCR5 will bind to RANTES, MIP-1α and MIP-1β and is predomi-nantly expressed on monocytes and T-cells. These three chemokines have been found to act as natural suppressors of HIV infection. In primary macrophages, it has been found that CD4 is necessary, but not sufficient, for HIV entry into the cell. The other coreceptor for HIV infection has been shown to be CCR5. People that are heterozygous for a mutation in the CCR5 gene have been found to have a slower progression to AIDS. People that are homozygous for the mutation are highly resistant to infection with the HIV virus.

The final presentation of the session described studies using mice carrying a targeted null mutation of the gene encoding inducible nitric oxide synthase to define the role of iNOS in in-flammatory responses. John Mudgett (Merck) first described the preparation of the iNOS-targeted mice in which the first four exons of the iNOS gene were removed by homologous recombination. Homozygous iNOS-deficient mice were viable, fertile and appeared phenotypic-ally normal through at least 14 months of age. In an acute model of systemic sepsis, anesthetized iNOS-deficient mice showed increased survival compared to wild-type controls. This enhanced survival was not observed for nonanesthetized mice.

Strikingly, iNOS-deficiency had no detectable impact on several mouse models of chronic inflammatory disease. For example, in collagen-induced arthritis, iNOS-deficient mice developed joint disease in a manner similar to control animals. This was not the case for IL-1β-deficient mice which were resistant to disease in this model. In the experimental autoimmune encephalo-myelitis (EAE) model of multiple sclerosis, iNOS-deficient mice appeared to develop somewhat more severe disease than wild-type littermates. The iNOS-targeted animals showed lower levels of disease remission than did the control animals. This effect on disease remission appeared to underlie the finding of more severe disease in the iNOS-deficient animals. In general, these studies using iNOS-deficient mice suggested that the deficiency produced a detectable phenotype more prominently in models of acute injury and inflammation, with minimal to no effect on models of chronic inflammation.

AAS 49
Therapeutic Strategies for Modulating the Inflammatory Diseases
© 1998 Birkhäuser Verlag Basel/Switzerland

ICE family proteases in inflammation and apoptosis

W.W. Wong

BASF Bioresearch Corporation, 100 Research Drive, Worcester, MA, 01605-4314, USA

Summary. The interleukin-1β converting enzyme (ICE) was first identified as a unique cysteine protease that processes the inactive precursor of the pro-inflammatory cytokine IL-1β to its mature active form. Subsequent revelation that a *C. elegans* cell death gene ced-3 bears sequence homology to ICE has led to rapid identification of at least nine other members of this gene family in humans, some of which are involved in apoptosis. Analyses of ICE-deficient mice generated by gene targeting technology reveal that this enzyme is important in maturation of several cytokines. The ICE deficient mice are resistant in several models of localized and systemic inflammation. ICE itself, however, is not required for Fas-mediated apoptosis, a physiological process for elimination of activated lymphocytes. Selective inhibitors of ICE would be novel therapeutic agents for treatment of diseases where excess inflammation contributes to pathological processes.

ICE family proteases

The interleukin-1β converting enzyme (ICE) was the first described member of a novel family of intracellular cysteine proteases with key roles in cytokine maturation and programmed cell death [1, 2]. To date, a total of ten human homologues have been identified in the tagged sequence database of human expressed genes (ETS). Based on sequence alignment, these proteases can be divided into three subfamilies. The ICE subfamily contains ICE, Tx/ICH-2/ICE$_{rel}$II, and ICE$_{rel}$III/Ty, the CPP32 subfamily contains CPP32/Apopain/Yama, Mch2, Mch-3/ICE-LAP-3/CMH-1, Mch4, FLICE/MACH/Mch5, and the ICH-1 subfamily contains ICH-1 and ICE-LAP-6 (Fig. 1) [3–14]. The degree of homology between subgroups averages about 30% while the members within each group are more similar, with sequence homologies ranging from 50% between CPP32 and Mch-2 to over 90% between Tx/ICH-2/ICE$_{rel}$II and ICE$_{rel}$III/Ty. A unifying family name, caspase, for cysteine/cytoplasmic- aspartate-specific-proteases, has been proposed, with individual family members numbered by order of discovery.

The proteases are all synthesized as proenzymes that range in size from 30 kDa to 45 kDa, with N-terminal prodomains that vary in size from about 30 amino acids to over 100 residues. In FLICE/MACH and Mch-4, the large prodomains encode death domain motifs and these structures are required for transmission of receptor-mediated death signals through interaction with receptor and adaptor molecules that contain similar motifs [11–13]. The prodomains of ICE, ICH-2, and ICH-1 may be similarly responsible for enzyme localization. Proteolytic removal of the N-terminal domain and, in some cases, a small linker peptide, produces two subunits of

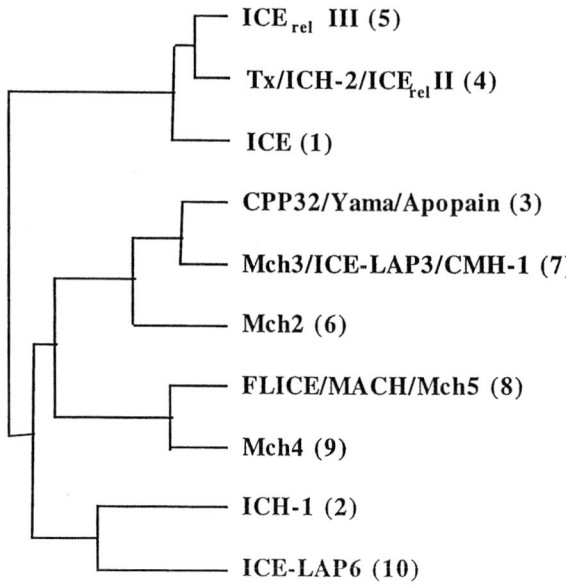

Figure 1. A dendrogram of the known human ICE-like proteases created by sequence alignment using PILEUP in GCG with gap weight of 3.0 and gap length weight of 0.1. The caspase designations are listed in parentheses.

approximately 18 kDa and 11 kDa that constitute the catalytically active heterodimer of each enzyme [2]. Crystallographic analyses indicate that the tertiary and quaternary structures of the catalytic domains of ICE and CPP32 are very similar [15–17]. Each heterodimer contains a dominant central six-strand β-sheet surrounded by five α-helices, and the holoenzyme contains two heterodimers aligned side-by-side along a two-fold axis of geometry. All caspases contain the signature motifs QACXG and SHG surrounding the catalytic cysteine and histidine and analogous Arg 179, Arg 349, Gln 283, and Ser 339 residues that define the S1 pocket, hence all have nearly absolute requirements for aspartate in the P1 position of their substrates [15–17]. The N-termini of subunits in all active enzymes begin with a residue that follows an Asp in the coding sequence, suggesting that activation involves auto-proteolysis or trans-activation by another member of the same family.

The substrate binding sites of ICE and CPP32 are grooves on the surfaces to which their respective tetrapeptide aldehyde inhibitors bind in an extended conformation. In each case, the side chain of P1 Asp reaches into a central depression of the enzyme to form strong ionic interactions with the surrounding residues that define the S1 pocket, and the aldehyde was observed as a thiohemiketal intermediate with the catalytic Cys 285. Residues from both subunits of ICE contribute to binding of the peptide substrate, especially with respect to the aspartyl side chain in P1. The amide backbone of Arg 341 and Ser 339 form hydrogen bonds with the amide backbone of their substrates in the P2 and P3 positions. The side chains of these residues in the substrates are orientated towards solvent, consistent with tolerance for broad substitutions in these positions in their respective peptide substrates [15–17]. ICE and CPP32 differ in their P4 specificities. CPP32 prefers Asp over Tyr in both substrate and peptidic inhibitors (Ki of Ac-DEVD-CHO=0.5 nM, Ki of Ac-YVAD-CHO=12 μM), while ICE prefers Tyr (Ki of Ac-YVAD-CHO=0.8 nM) but tolerates Asp (Ki of Ac-DEVD-CHO=9 nM) [18]. These preferences were consistent with the significant differences observed in the architecture of the S4 subsites of these two enzymes. The S4 region in ICE is wide and shallow, easily accommodating bulky hydrophobic side chains such as that of Tyr, while tolerating the side chain of Asp. The analogous region in CPP32 is narrower with several residues forming a complex network of hydrogen bonds with the side chain of Asp at P4 [15–17]. An extra loop of ten amino acids, starting at Glu 248 in CPP32, is an added feature of members of this subfamily that provides further interaction with P4 and confers additional substrate specificity at this site [17]. Further analysis of the three-dimensional structure of other enzymes in this family should reveal structural features that support their fine specificities for macromolecular substrates.

Of the other known caspases, Mch3 is most homologous to CPP32 and exhibits a similar preference for substrates and inhibitors containing the -DEVD-X sequence. It is also well-established as a downstream effector protease, and may function redundantly with CPP32 in apoptosis. Mch2 has been proposed in the literature to be a Lamin A-cleaving and CPP32-activating protease in apoptosis [19]. Substrate specificity studies show that Mch2 prefers β-branched amino acids in the substrate P4 position. This explains efficient cleavage of Lamin A by Mch2, where cleavage occurs at VEID-N, and is consistent with CPP32 maturation at the cleavage site IETD-S. The substrate specificities ICH-2 resembles that of ICE, preferring hydrophobic or β-branched residues in P4.

Intracellular ICE exists primarily as its p45 precursor form, suggesting that the mature, active enzyme decays rapidly. Recombinant ICE has a half life of less than ten minutes *in vitro*, and loss of activity is associated with decay from tetramer to dimer and degradation of the 10 kDa subunit. Treatment of recombinant enzyme with the peptide aldehyde inhibitor Ac-YVAD-CHO, followed by its removal, enhances the stability of the tetrameric enzyme [20]. Further oligomeric stability is conferred when Asp 381, a site for autoproteolytic degradation, is converted to Glu [21]. Such stabilization of enzyme activity through substrate interaction may be relevant and important in the regulation of the intracellular levels of ICE. In the absence of its native substrate, pro-IL-1β, ICE would not accumulate in cells and lead to unnecessary apoptosis. By contrast, CPP32 remains as a stable tetramer *in vitro* even in the absence of substrate or substrate analogs. The ease with which subunits of CPP32 can be detected in cell lysates during apoptotic events is consistent with its observed stability *in vitro,* and its *in vivo* role in cellular suicide. Upon activation of CPP32, the cell death program may be well past commitment and no further check-point is warranted.

ICE in inflammation

ICE-deficient mice generated by gene-targeting technology provided a means to evaluate the role of ICE in cytokine production and inflammatory responses, using a variety of *ex vivo* and *in vivo* approaches. Disruption of the targeted gene was confirmed by DNA analysis and corresponding absence of ICE mRNA and ICE protein from isolated tissues of homozygous ICE -/- mice [22, 23]. In *ex vivo* experiments, the peritoneal macrophages from these mice lacked the capacity to process and secrete mature IL-1β upon stimulation by LPS and ATP, although synthesis of pro-IL-1β was normal. This resulted in the intracellular accumulation of the inactive cytokine precursor. Suprisingly, a parallel decrease in the processing of IL-1α from its precursor to about 25% of its normal level was also observed [22]. Pro-IL-1α itself is not a substrate for ICE, and previous evidence had suggested that a calcium-activated neutral proteases (CANP) may be involved in its activation [24]. An indirect role for ICE in IL-1α maturation was confirmed when cotransfection of the cDNA that encoded ICE and pro-IL-1α into COS-1 cells resulted in the release of mature IL-α. Enzymatically active ICE was required: cotransfection with the cDNA of ICE lacking the catalytic cysteine did not lead to release of IL-1α. Addition of AK295, a dipeptide ketoamide inhibitor specific for calpain-like proteases but not ICE blocked this process. Radio-sequencing of the released IL-1α produced [35]Met in the ninth cycle, consistent with an N-terminal sequence produced by the proteolytic cleavage of the precursor after Phe 118 [25]. Partial blockade of IL-α can be achieved in LPS-stimulated human peripheral blood monocytic cells by Ac-YVAD-aldehyde, an inhibitor specific for ICE, at concentrations that completely blocked the production of mature IL-β. These observations suggest that an ICE-dependent mechanism exists for IL-1α maturation in human cells as well [25]. Potential mechanisms for ICE-activation of a calpain-like protease may include conversion of zymogen to active protease by proteolytic removal of a prodomain, or inactivation of an endogenous inhibitor such as calpastatin.

ICE-deficient animals also provided a model to evaluate the impact of the absence of functional protease on a variety of inflammatory responses. When these mice were injected with 800 μg of LPS intravenously, the circulating levels of plasma IL-1β and IL-1α were 5% and 25% of the respective levels seen in their wild-type littermate controls. Under these conditions, the level of TNF-α in these animals were comparable to the wild-type controls, but there was significant reduction in the levels of IFN-γ and IL-6. These effects may be secondary to the decrease in IL-1 levels. Reduction in the composite cytokine response had a dramatic impact: at least 70% of the ICE deficient animals survived the lethal effect of high-dose LPS, compared to no survival in the ICE-sufficient animals [22]. Knock-out mice lacking a functional IL-1β gene showed a decrease in the plasma levels of only IL-1β after administration of high-dose LPS, and these mice were susceptible to the lethal effects of high dose LPS treatment [26]. Reconstitution of ICE -/- mice by addition of IL-1β did not restore their susceptibility to high dose LPS treatment. Therefore the resistance in this model may be attributed to down regulation of additional cytokines such as IL-1α, and further suggest that ICE inhibitors may be beneficial in the treatment of septic shock. ICE is also important in localized responses to LPS: ICE -/- mice showed significant reduction in LPS-induced foot pad edema. The potential effects of ICE blockade in ischemia-induced neuroinflammatory responses was also evaluated in a model in which ICE -/- mice were subjected to occlusion of the middle cerebral artery. The ischemic hemisphere exhibited a significant decrease in the necrotic lesion relative to wild type control mice [27]. Inhibition of ICE represents an approach in which the levels of several cytokines can be modulated simultaneously, and offers greater therapeutic impact in the treatment of a variety of inflammatory diseases.

ICE and ICE-like proteases in apoptosis

ICE was suspected to be involved in apoptosis when it was discovered that its sequence was homologous to the *C. elegans* cell death gene *ced-3* and overexpression of murine ICE in fibroblasts led to apoptosis of the transfected cells [28]. Apoptotic death of neuronal cells as a consequence of nerve growth factor withdrawal was blocked by expression of crmA [29], a serpin-like protein inhibitor of ICE derived from the cowpox virus. These findings raised concerns for our drug discovery efforts because chronic treatment with an ICE inhibitor may block physiological apoptosis and induce undesirable effects such as neoplasms and autoimmune syndromes. Evidence for defects in physiological apoptosis was sought in the ICE-deficient mice. These mice developed normally, appeared healthy and were fertile. Gross and histopathological examinations revealed no abnormalities in all major organs. Unlike the p53 -/- animals, there has been no evidence for spontaneous development of tumors even at up to eighteen months of age [22].

Although dexamethasone and gamma-irradiation induced apoptosis were normal in thymocytes from ICE -/- animals [22, 23], partial resistance of these cells to Fas-induced apoptosis, a process required for elimination of activated lymphocytes, was reported in one study [23]. Careful examination of all parameters relating to Fas-induced events *in vivo* have revealed no defects in the ICE -/- mice. The distribution of B-cells, CD4+ and CD8+ T-cell subsets in thymuses, spleens and lymph nodes, were normal and no anti-DNA antibodies were found in their sera.

These mice demonstrated no symptoms of lymphadenopathy and lymphoproliferative diseases similar to those found in the *MRL-lpr* or the *gld* strains with respective defects in Fas and Fas ligand. The effect of Fas-induced hepatic cell death was also investigated in these mice and they were equally susceptible to lethality induced by treatment with anti-Fas antibodies as their wild-type controls. Our collective results in the ICE deficient mice did not reveal a significant role for ICE in Fas-mediated apoptosis *in vivo*. Such discordance between *in vitro* and *in vivo* findings may indicate the limitations of cell-based experiments performed with single time points. If the kinetics of the death program was merely delayed but not actually blocked in the *in vitro* experiments, then a major *in vivo* impact would not be expected. In studies which addressed the potential role of ICE in CTL-mediated killing, embryonic fibroblasts and B lymphocytes from ICE -/- mice were resistant to Granzyme-B-mediated apoptosis [30]. The physiological consequence of these findings are yet to be determined.

Since the early reports implicating ICE in apoptosis, a plethora of studies have appeared supporting dominant roles for caspases in apoptotic events. The ability of the baculovirus anti-apoptotic protein, p35, to block multiple caspases from nematodes to mammals further highlights their central and conserved role in programmed cell death [31, 32]. In suicide pathways triggered by physiological ligands such as Fas or TNF-α, signals from the receptors are transmitted through one or more adaptor proteins such as FADD and TRADD that contain death domain motifs. These membrane-proximal protein-protein interactions can be modulated by the 'inactivators of apoptosis' (iaps) [33, 34]. The first caspase family member to be activated through death domain interaction is FLICE/MACH/Mch5 [11, 12]. Mch4 also contains a death domain motif in its prodomain and may be activated in analogous fashion through other cell surface receptors [12]. In turn, the receptor-proximal proteases activate several other caspases in a proteolytic cascade: Mch-2 followed by Mch-3 and CPP32. Susceptibility of Fas-induced apoptosis to inhibition by crmA, a serpin that inactivates ICE 10,000 fold faster than CPP32, and detection of proteolytic activity for Ac-YVAD-AMC substrate early in lysates of Fas-activated cells further suggest that activation of an additional ICE-like protease occurs prior to CPP32/Mch-3 activation. By contrast, stress or drug induced death programs are resistant to crmA inhibition. These signals probably by-pass the upstream proteases, and directly activate the effector proteases by yet unidentified mechanisms [35].

The death proteases exert their detrimental effects not only by destruction of the structural elements and vital repair mechanisms, but their effects can be further amplified through activation of other enzymes such as kinases. One of the substrates of a CPP32-like enzyme is PKC-δ, the cleavage and activation of which results in a hyperactive catalytic domain that induces morphological phenotype characteristic of apoptotic cells upon transfection into HeLa cells [36]. Thus, inhibitors of caspases are attractive targets for therapeutic intervention in diseases which result from excess or inappropriate apoptosis. However, the benefits of such inhibitors would rely on the selection of a molecular target that is critical to initiation of apoptosis. As the specificities of caspases may be redundant, and many different enzymes may orchestrate the destructive events, selective inhibition of an effector protease that is too far downstream may not produce the desired therapeutic impact.

A parallel proteolytic cascade has been proposed for activation of the ICE-mediated cytokine processing. Cotransfection of ICE cDNA and a murine gene encoding a protease homologous to human ICH-2 or ICE $_{rel}$III resulted in the enhanced capacity of ICE to process pro-IL-1β [37]. Human ICH-2, but not CPP32, Mch-3, Mch-2 or ICH-1, can process pro-IL-1β at reduced efficiency [4]. Because of the high homology to ICH-2, we predict that ICE $_{rel}$III /Ty will have similar overlapping specificity with ICE. These three proteases may represent a distinct branch of the caspase family with roles in maturation of other proinflammatory cytokines or hormones. Inhibitors of these enzymes may have therapeutic applications in multiple disorders.

References

1. Cerretti, D.P., Kozlosky, C.J., Mosley, B., Nelson, N., Van, N.K., Greenstreet, T.A., March, C.J., Kronheim, S.R., Druck, T., Cannizzaro, L.A., Huebner, K. and Black, R.A. (1992) Molecular cloning of the interleukin-1β converting enzyme. *Science* 256: 97–100.
2. Thornberry, N.A., Bull, H.G., Calaycay, J.R., Chapman, K.T., Howard, A.D., Kostura, M.J., Miller, D.K., Molineaux, S.M., Weidner, J.R., Aunins, J., Elliston, K.O., Ayala, J.M., Casano, F.J., Chin, J., Ding, G.J.-F., Egger, L.A., Gaffney, E.P., Limjuco, G., Palyha, O.C., Raju, S.M., Rolando, A.M., Salley, J.P., Yamin, T.-T., Lee, T.D., Shively, J.E., MacCross, M., Mumford, R.A., Schmidt, J.A. and Tocci, M.J. (1992) novel hetero-dimeric cysteine protease is required for interleukin-1 beta processing in monocytes. *Nature* 356: 768–774.
3. Faucheu, C., Diu, A., Chan, A.W., Blanchet, A.M., Miossec, C., Herve, F., Collard-Dutilleul, V., Gu, Y., Aldape, R.A., Lippke, J.A. et al. (1995) A novel human protease similar to the interleukin-1 beta converting enzyme induces apoptosis in transfected cells. *EMBO J.* 14: 1914–1922.
4. Kamens, J., Paskind, M., Hugunin, M., Talanian, R.V., Allen, H., Banach, D., Bump, N., Hackett, M., Johnston, C.G., Li, P., Mankovich, J.A., Terranova. M. and Ghayur, T. (1995) Identification and characterization of ICH-2, a novel member of the interleukin 1 β-converting enzyme family of cysteine proteases. *J. Biol. Chem.* 270: 15250–15256.
5. Munday, N.A., Vaillancourt, J.P., Ali, A., Casano, F.J., Miller, D.K., Molineaux, S.M., Yamin, T., Yu, V.L. and Nicholson, D.W. (1995) Molecular cloning and pro-apoptotic activity of ICE (rel) II and ICE (rel) III, members of the ICE/CED-3 family of cysteine proteases. *J. Biol. Chem.* 270: 15870–15876.
6. Fernandes-Alnemri, T., Litwack, G. and Alnemri, E.S. (1994) CPP32, a novel human apoptotic protein with homology to *Caenorhabditis elegans* cell death protein Ced-3 and mammalian interleukin-1β-converting enzyme. *J. Biol. Chem.* 269: 30761–30764.
7. Wang, L., Miura, M., Bergeron, L., Zhu, H. and Yuan, J.Y. (1994) Ich-1, an ICE/ced-3-related gene, encodes both positive and negative regulators of programmed cell death. *Cell* 78: 739–750.
8. Kumar, S., Kinoshita, M., Noda, M., Copeland N.G. and Jenkins, N.A. (1994) Induction of apoptosis by the mouse Nedd2 gene, which encodes a protein similar to the product of the *Caenorhabditis elegans* cell death gene ced-3 and the mammalian IL-1 beta-converting enzyme. *Gene Develop.* 8: 1613–1626.
9. Fernandes-Alnemri, T., Litwack, G. and Alnemri, E.S. (1995) Mch2, a new member of the apoptotic Ced-3/ice cysteine protease gene family. *Cancer Res.* 55: 2737–2742.
10. Fernandes-Alnemri, T., Takahashi, A., Armstrong, R., Krebs, J., Fritz, L., Tomaselli, K.J., Wang, L., Yu, Z., Croce, C.M., Salveson, G., Earnshaw, W.C., Litwack, G. and Alnemri, E.S. (1995) Mch3, a novel human apoptotic cysteine protease highly related to CPP32. *Cancer Res.* 55: 6045–6052.
11. Muzio, M., Chinnaiyan, A.M., Kischkel, F.C., O'Rourke, K., Shevchenko, A., Ni, J., Scaffidi, C., Bretz, J.D., Zhang, M., Gentz, R., Mann, M., Krammer, P.H., Peter, M.E. and Dixit, V.M. (1996) FLICE, a novel FADD-

homologous ICE/CED-3-like protease, is recruited to the CD95 (Fas/APO-1) death-inducing signaling complex. *Cell* 85: 817–27.
12. Boldin, M.P., Goncharov, T.M., Goltsev, Y.V. and Wallach, D. (1996) Involvement of MACH, a novel MORT1/FADD-interacting protease, in Fas/APO-1- and TNF receptor-induced cell death. *Cell* 85: 803–15.
13. Fernandes-Alnemri, T., Armstrong, R.C., Krebs, J., Srinivasula, S.M., Wang, L., Bullrich, F., Fritz, L.C., Trapani, J.A., Tomaselli, K.J., Litwack, G., Alnemri, E.S. (1996) *In vitro* activation of CPP32 and Mch3 by Mch4, a novel human apoptotic cysteine protease containing two FADD-like domains. *Proc. Natl. Acad. Sci. USA* 93: 7464–7469.
14. Duan, H., Orth, K., Chinnaiyan, A.M., Poirier, G.G., Froelich, C.J., He, W.W. and Dixit, V.M. (1996) ICE-LAP6, a novel member of the ICE/Ced-3 gene family, is activated by the cytotoxic T-cell protease granzyme B. *J. Biol. Chem.* 271: 16720–16724.
15. Walker, N.P.C., Talanian, R.V., Brady, K.D., Dang, L.C., Bump, N.J., Ferenz, C.R., Franklin, S., Ghayur, T., Hackett, M.C., Hammill, L.D., Herzog, L., Hugunin, M., Houy, W., Mankovich, J.A., Mcguiness, L., Orlewicz, E., Paskind, M., Pratt, C.A., Reis, P., Summani, A., Terranova, M., Welch, J.P., Xiong, L., Moller, A., Tracey, D.E., Kamen, R. and Wong, W.W. (1994) Crystal structure of the cysteine protease interleukin-1 beta-converting enzyme: A (p20/p10)(2) homodimer. *Cell* 78: 343–352.
16. Wilson, K.P., Black, J.A.F., Thomson, J.A., Kim, E.E., Griffith, J.P., Navia, M.A., Murcko, M.A., Chambers, S.P., Aldape, R.A., Raybuck, S.A. and Livingston, D.J. (1994) Structure and mechanism of interleukin-1 beta converting enzyme. *Nature* 370: 270–275.
17. Rotonda, J., Nicholson, D.W., Fazil, K.M., Gallant, M., Gareau, Y., Labelle, M., Peterson, E.P., Rasper, D.M., Ruel, R., Vaillancourt, J.P., Thornberry, N.A. and Becker, J.W. (1996) The three-dimensional structure of apopain/CPP32, a key mediator of apoptosis. *Nature Struct. Biol.* 3: 619–25.
18. Nicholson, D.W., Ali, A., Thornberry, N.A., Vaillancourt, J.P., Ding, C.K., Gallant, M., Gareau, Y., Griffin, P.R., Labelle, M., Lazebnik, Y.A. et al. (1995) Identification and inhibition of the ICE/CED-3 protease necessary for mammalian apoptosis. *Nature* 376: 37–43.
19. Orth, K., Chinnaiyan, A.M., Garg, M., Froelich, C.J. and Dixit, V.M. (1996) The CED-3/ICE-like protease Mch2 is activated during apoptosis and cleaves the death substrate lamin A. *J. Biol. Chem.* 271: 16443–6.
20. Talanian, R.V., Dang, L.C., Ferenz, C.R., Hackett, M.C., Mankovich, J.A., Welch, J.P., Wong, W.W. and Brady, K.D. (1996) Stability and oligomeric equilibria of refolded interleukin-1 beta converting enzyme. *J. Biol. Chem.* 271: 21853–21858.
21. Dang, L.C., Talanian, R.V., Banach, D., Hackett, M.C., Gilmore, J.L., Hays, S.J., Mankovich, J.A. and Brady, K.D. (1996) Preparation of an autolysis-resistant Interleukin-1β Converting Enzyme mutant. *Biochemistry* 35: 14910–14916.
22. Li, P., Allen, H., Banerjee, S., Franklin, S., Herzog, L., Johnston, C., McDowell, J., Paskind, M., Rodman, L., Salfeld, J., Towne, E., Tracey, D., Wardwell, S., Wei, F.-Y., Wong, W., Kamen, R. and Seshadri, T. (1995) Mice deficient in interleukin-1β converting enzyme (ICE) are defective in production of mature interleukin-1β (IL-1 β) and resistant to endotoxic shock. *Cell* 80: 401–411.
23. Kuida, K., Lippke, J.A., Ku, G., Harding, M.W., Livingston, D.J., Su, M.S.-S. and Flavell, R.A. (1995) Altered cytokine export and apoptosis in mice deficient in interleukin-1 beta converting enzyme. *Science* 267: 2000–2003.
24. Kobayashi, y. Yamamoto, K., Saido, T., Kawasaki, H., Oppenheim, J.J. and Matsushima, K. (1990) Identification of calcium activated neutral protease as a processing enzyme of human interleukin 1 α. *Proc. Natl. Acad. Sci. USA* 87: 5548–5552.
25. Herzog, L., Ferenz, C.R., Paskind, M., Hugunin, M., Ghayur, T., Wardwell, S., Seshadri, T., Li, P., Kamen, R., Wong, W., Tracey, D. and Allen, H. (1996) Interleukin 1β Converting Enzyme stimulates calpain-mediated production of mature IL-1α. *J. Biol. Chem.*; *submitted for publication.*
26. Shornick, L.P., De, T.P., Mariathasan, S., Goellner, J., Strauss, S.J., Karr, R.W., Ferguson, T.A. and Chaplin, D.D. (1996) Mice deficient in IL-1 beta manifest impaired contact hypersensitivity to trinitrochlorobenzone. *J. Exp. Med.* 183: 1427–36.
27. Betz, A.L., Schielke, G.P. and Yang, G.-Y. (1996) Interleukin-1 in cerebral ischemia. *Keio J. Med.*; *in press.*
28. Yuan, J., Shaham, S., Ledoux, S., Ellis, H.M. and Horvitz, H.R. (1993) The *C. elegans* cell death gene *ced-3* encodes a protein similar to mammalian Interleukin-1β-Converting Enzyme. *Cell* 75: 641–652.
29. Gagliardini, V., Fernandez, P.A., Lee, R.K., Drexler, H.C., Rotello, R.J., Fishman, M.C. and Yuan, J. (1994) Prevention of vertebrate neuronal death by the crmA gene. *Science* 263: 826–828.
30. Shi, L., Chen, G., MacDonald, G., Bergeron, L., Li, H., Miura, M., Rotello, R.J., Miller, D.K., Li, P., Seshadri, T., Yuan, J. and Greenberg, A.H. (1996) Activation of an interleukin 1 converting enzyme-dependent apoptosis pathway by granzyme B. *Proc. Natl. Acad. Sci. USA* 93: 11002–11006.
31. Bump, N.J., Hackett, M., Hugunin, M., Seshagiri, S., Brady, K., Chen, P., Ferenz, C., Franklin, S., Ghayur, T., Li, P., Licari, P., Mankovich, J., Shi, L.F., Greenberg, A.H., Miller, L.K. and Wong, W.W. (1995) Inhibition of ICE family proteases by baculovirus antiapoptotic protein p35. *Science* 269: 1885–1888.
32. Xue, D. and Horvitz, H.R. (1995) Inhibition of the *Caenorhabditis elegans* cell-death protease CED-3 by a CED-3 cleavage site in baculovirus p35 protein. *Nature* 377: 248–251.
33. Rothe, M., Pan, M.-G., Henzel, W.J., Ayres, T.M. and Goeddel, D.V. (1995) TRAF2-mediated activation of NF-kappa B by TNF receptor 2 and CD40. *Cell* 83: 1243–1252.

34. Liston, P., Roy, N., Tamai, K., Lefebvre, C., Baird, S., Cherton-Horvat, G., Farahani, R., McLean, M., Ikeda, J.-E., MacKenzie, A. and Korneluk, R.G. (1996) Suppression of apoptosis in mammalian cells by NAIP and a related family of IAP genes. *Nature* 379: 349–353.
35. Chinnaiyan, A.M., Orth, K., O'Rourke, K., Duan, H., Poirier, G.G. and Dixit, V.M. (1996) Molecular ordering of the cell death pathway. *J. Biol. Chem.* 271: 4573–4576.
36. Ghayur, T., Hugunin, M., Datta, R., Ratnofsky, S., Wong, W. and Kufe, D. (1996) Proteolytic activation of protein kinase C delta by an ICE/CED-3-like protease induces characteristics of apoptosis. *J. Exp. Med.* 184: 2399–2404.
37. Wang, S., Miura, M., Jung, Y., Zhu, H., Gagliardini, V., Shi, L., Greenberg, A.H. and Yuan, J. (1996) Identification and characterization of Ich-3, a member of the interleukin-1β converting enzyme (ICE)/Ced-3 family and an upstream regulator of ICE. *J. Biol. Chem.* 271: 20580–20587.

AAS 49
Therapeutic Strategies for Modulating the Inflammatory Diseases
© 1998 Birkhäuser Verlag Basel/Switzerland

Molecular mechanisms of costimulation

S.C. Gilman[1] and R.J. Noelle[2]

[1]*Pfizer Inc., Eastern Point Rd, Groton, CT 06371, USA*
[2]*Department of Microbiology, Dartmouth Medical School, Lebanon, NH 03756, USA*

The Immunology Symposium at the 7th Annual Meeting focused on the role of co-stimulatory molecules in the regulation of humoral and cell-mediated immunity. Primarily studies have focused on the role of two sets of receptor-ligand pairs. These are CD28/CTLA4 and their co-receptors B7-1 and B7-2 as well as CD40 and its ligand, gp39 (CD4OL). It is clear from the data presented that these molecules represent very attractive therapeutic targets for clinical intervention in autoimmune disease and in graft rejection.

Dr. Randy Noelle (Dartmouth Medical School) presented a summary of the work that has emerged in the area of CD40 and its ligand in humoral and cell-mediated immunity. While it was clear that this ligand-receptor pair is critical in humoral immunity, it also appears to play a central role in the area of T-cell priming and expansion. Studies showing the role of gp39 in acute graft *vs.* host disease and in graft rejection all point to gp39 as a major player in the regulation of cell-mediated immune responses.

Dr. Marc Jenkins (University of Minnesota) provided some vivid insights into the parameters that govern the *in vivo* expansion of antigen-specific T-cells. Using a system that has been pioneered by Dr. Jenkins, he showed that the expansion of T-cell receptor transgenic T-cells *in vivo* required antigen and co-stimulation *via* the B7-CD28 axis. In addition, a major effort was exerted to try to understand why adjuvants are so critical for T-cell expansion. Using the technology Dr. Jenkins has been able to create a "cytokine cocktail" that begins to replace the need for adjuvants in inducing T-cell immunity.

Dr. Arlene Sharpe (Brigham and Woman's Hospital) presented studies in a series of genetically-deficient mice that unequivicolly demonstrated the function of co-stimulatory molecules in development of humoral and cell-mediated immune responses. Targeted deletion of both B7-1 and B7-2 largely ablated primary and secondary humoral immune responses, suggesting that there are no other co-stimulatory molecules that can significantly compensate for the loss of these costimulatory molecules. In addition, a series of studies in the CTLA4-deficient mouse revealed that CTLA4 is a profound negative regulator of immunity by virtue of the fact that the CTLA-4 deficient mice die early in life from massive, multisystemic immunoinflammatory disease.

Dr. Jeffrey Bluestone (University of Chicago) presented studies which directly tested the efficacy of CTLA4-Ig as an immunosuppressive agent for the prevention of kidney allograft rejection in monkeys. The data presented showed that CTLA4-Ig could lengthen the time of allograft survival in outbred rhesus monkeys. In addition, Dr. Bluestone presented studies that underscored the importance of the temporal role of co-stimulatory molecules in the regulation of the immune responses. Within the context of B7-1 and B7-2, he demonstrated that the time at which these molecules were blocked could qualitatively influence the course of the ensuing immune response.

Taken together, these presentations provided an exciting picture of the future of these molecules as superb therapeutic targets for the management of inappropriate immune responses.

AAS 49
Therapeutic Strategies for Modulating the Inflammatory Diseases
© 1998 Birkhäuser Verlag Basel/Switzerland

CD40 and its ligand in cell-mediated immunity

R.J. Noelle

Department of Microbiology, Dartmouth Medical School, Lebanon, NH 03756, USA

Summary. CD40 and its ligand (gp39, CD40L, TBAM) is central to the control of thymus-dependent humoral immunity. However, in recent years it has become evident that CD40 signaling also is critical in the development of cell-mediated immune responses. How CD40 regulates cell-mediated immunity is discussed.

Introduction

CD40, a mitogenic receptor expressed on all mature B lymphocytes [1, 2], is a member of the nerve growth factor receptor (NGFR) family of receptors [3]. The ligand for CD40, gp39 is a type II membrane protein which is homologous to TNF-α and -β [4, 5] other NGFR family ligands. Evidence that CD40 is an important mitogenic receptor on B-cells is derived from studies that show highly efficient triggering of human B-cells by anti-CD40 and co-factors such as anti-CD20, anti-Ig and lymphokines [4–9]. In the presence of these co-factors, anti-CD40, has been shown to initiate both B-cell growth and differentiation. Similar to anti-CD40, gp39, expressed as a recombinant membrane protein or a soluble protein also activates B-cells in the presence of co-stimulators [4, 10].

gp39 is transiently expressed on activated CD4+ T_h cells *in vitro* and is induced *in vivo* on CD4+ T-cells as a result of antigen administration [11]. The CD4+ T-cell population expressing gp39 *in vivo* have been localized *in situ* juxtaposed to B-cells producing antibodies to the immunizing antigen. *In vitro* and *in vivo* data suggest that during the course of cognate T_h-B interaction, transient expression of gp39 by CD4+ T-cells is the result of antigen-presentation [12]. Once expressed, gp39 binds to CD40 and reciprocally triggers B-cell activation. The ability of a mAb specific for gp39, MR1, to block the capacity of gp39-bearing T_h to activate B-cells *in vitro* has implicated gp39 as an important molecule in T-cell-dependent B-cell activation, as reviewed in [13].

Further evidence implicating gp39-CD40 involvement in humoral immune responses has recently been provided by several groups demonstrating that mutations in the gene encoding gp39 result in the inability of humans to respond to TD antigens, as reviewed in [13]. An immunodeficiency characterized by failure to mount TD humoral immune responses, Hyper-IgM syndrome (HIM), results in the expression of a defective gp39 molecule which lacks CD40 binding capacity. Although the B lymphocytes from these patients are reported to be normal mutations in the gp39 molecule interrupt B-cell triggering through CD40 and subsequent B-cell activation and immunoglobulin production. Over the past 3 years, insights into the function of gp39 and CD40 in the regulation of humoral immunity have been provided by studies in gp39- [14, 15] and CD40-deficient [16] mice and in mice treated with anti-gp39 [11, 17, 18]. For the most part, all of these systems agree that gp39 interactions are essential for secondary immune responses to TD antigens and in the formation of GC. Studies using anti-gp39 [18] or a soluble form of CD40 [19] to inhibit the *in vivo* function of gp39 showed that the generation of memory B-cells is also dependent on this ligand-receptor pair.

CD40 triggers B-cells to become mature, competent APCs

Parker and Eynon [20] demonstrated that an antigen targeted to resting B-cells which inadequately crosslinked sIg was presented to T-cells in a manner which resulted in antigen specific T-cell anergy. From these studies they proposed that presentation of antigen by resting B-cells to virgin T-cells, in the absence of sufficient levels of B7-1, results in the induction of T-cell anergy. Harding and Allison also showed that CTL responses to an allogeneic tumor cell line, P815 required that the tumor cells be transfected with the gene encoding B7-1 [21]. Although there is compelling evidence that resting B-cells may induce tolerance under specific conditions [20], the general use of B-cells as vehicles to induce peripheral T-cell tolerance to a wide spectrum of antigens has not materialized. One explanation for why allogeneic resting B-cells are not universal inducers of tolerance induction is that upon administration to the allogeneic host, the B-cells are activated by alloreactive T-cells. As a consequence of this inadvertent activation, the allogeneic B-cells are stimulated, express heightened levels of B7 family members and *immunize* the host. We have shown that if B-cell activation is blocked by anti-gp39, allogeneic B-cells are superb inducers of tolerance under a variety of conditions.

To test the hypothesis that antigen-bearing B-cells could induce tolerance in the presence of anti-gp39, B-cells were prepared from C57BL/6 (H-2^b) mice and injected into Balb/c (H-2^d) mice. Some groups received anti-gp39 (250 µg/mouse/2 days) for 6 days at which point the spleens from these recipient animals were removed and used as effector cells in a standard cytotoxic T-cell assay. The results demonstrates that *in vivo* administration of allogeneic splenic B-cells and anti-gp39 results in hypo-responsiveness of alloantigen specific CTL activity and CD4$^+$ proliferative responses to alloantigen. Assessment of third party responses in the CTL and MLR assays confirms that the tolerogenic effect is allospecific. These data have been published [22]. Therefore, B-cells have to be triggered by CD40 before they become competent APC to trigger T-cell activation and generate effector T-cells.

The administration of B-cells into mice genetically deficient in gp39 induces T-cell tolerance

In lieu of using anti-gp39 to block the function of gp39, one would predict that the administration of allogenic B-cells into gp39 -/- mice [14] would induce allospecific tolerance. Indeed, the administration of allogeneic B-cells into gp39 -/- mice induce allospecific hyporesponsiveness of CD4 and CD8 T-cells. These observations confirm the results observed with anti-gp39 administration and show that in the absence of a CD40 signal, B-cells are tolerogenic.

The administration of B-cells and anti-gp39 can induce transplantation tolerance

In collaboration with David Parker, Aldo Rossini and Dale Greiner and co-workers at UMass, the tolerization regime of using allogeneic B-cells and anti-gp39 was applied to a system of transplantation tolerance, as published [23]. The purpose of this study was to ask if the unresponsiveness that was induced by allogenic B-cells and anti-gp39 was sufficiently profound to allow the transplant of allogenic pancreatic islet cells into tolerized mice. Thus, mice were induced to become diabetic by the chemical destruction of the endogenous islet cells, tolerized by the administration of allogeneic B-cells and anti-gp39 and then transplanted with allogeneic islets. Without any prior tolerization or simply by the administration of allogeneic B-cells, the mice rapidly rejected the allogeneic islet cells. The administration of anti-gp39 prolonged graft survival indefinitely in 40–50% of the mice. Virtually all of the transplanted mice pretreated with allogeneic B-cells and anti-gp39 retained the allogeneic grafts indefinitely. If the allogeneic B-cells and the allogeneic islet grafts were mismatched for the alloantigen, the success rate of graft survival dropped to that observed with anti-gp39 alone. These data, together with the data presented above, confirms that allogeneic B-cells, if deprived of the CD40 signal will induce T-cell unresponsiveness, and in this case, the tolerance was sufficiently profound to allow the transplant of an allograft.

All APC may require a CD40 signal so as to prime T-cells to alloantigen

While the observations with B-cells were somewhat anticipated based on their immature APC activity prior to CD40 signaling, the function of CD40 in stimulating professional APC to acquire co-stimulatory activity *in vivo* is less clear. Studies clearly show that some dendritic cells constitutively express costimulatory molecules and therefore, it was not necessarily anticipated that anti-gp39 administration would impede their ability to present alloantigen. These questions were addressed indirectly by asking whether acute graft vs host disease (aGVHD) was blocked by anti-gp39 administration. The hallmark feature of aGVHD is that the donor T-cells mount a CTL response against the F1 host alloantigens. Published studies have shown that anti-gp39 can block the generation of aGVHD in mice [24]. A brief treatment with anti-gp39 produced long-lived protection from aGVHD suggesting that even after the antibody disappeared from the periphery, no disease developed. In order to evaluate if T-cell unresponsiveness was induced as a consequence of anti-gp39 treatment, T-cells from GVHD mice that were treated with anti-gp39 were asked to transfer disease. No transfer of GHVD could be obtained from mice treated with anti-gp39, suggesting that the anti-gp39 resulted in T-cell tolerance. Alternative to using anti-gp39 to interfere with the development of GVHD, we have also shown that if T-cells from gp39 -/- mice were transferred into an F1 host, no indication of GVHD was noted. When WT parental T-cells were transferred into an F1, a profound reduction in splenic cellularity was obvious; however, when gp39 -/- T-cells were transferred no reduction in cellularity was noted. AGVHD typically is lethal to >95% of mice within 21 days. Indeed, the transfer of WT T-cells caused death in >95% of recipients. In those recipients receiving WT T-cells and anti-gp39 or gp39 -/- T-cells, >90% were alive with no signs of disease >50 days. Upon more extensive analysis of mice receiving gp39 -/- T-cells, minimal if any features of GVHD were observed. These data suggest that the host is inducing tolerance to host MHC molecules in the donor T-cell population. This implies that in the absence of the CD40 signal, host APC are tolerogenic and therefore would include host dendritic cells and macrophages. This observation raises the issue of whether professional APC (like dendritic cells and macrophages) need a CD40 signal to prime T-cells.

Direct evidence for a role of gp39 in T-cell expansion *in vivo* came from the work of Flavell and co-workers [25]. These investigators demonstrated that the expansion of gp39 -/- T-cell receptor transgenic T-cells was severely impaired when compared to WT controls. Although these experiments did not directly address the defect which caused the altered priming in ligand knockout mice, it is possible that a lack of gp39 signaling to the APC is a likely reason for poor T-cell expansion.

A model of CD40 regulation of T-cell activation

Taken together, our data can be assimilated into a model whereby CD40 signaling regulates T-cell activation. It is known that engagement of the TCR can induce the upregulation of gp39 (see Fig. 1). The result of gp39 upregulation is the triggering of CD40 on the APC. Engagement of CD40 has been shown to increase the expression of B7-1 and B7-2, as well as induce the upregulation of cytokines (e.g. IL-12) and chemokines (e.g. IL-8). Therefore, it appears that CD40

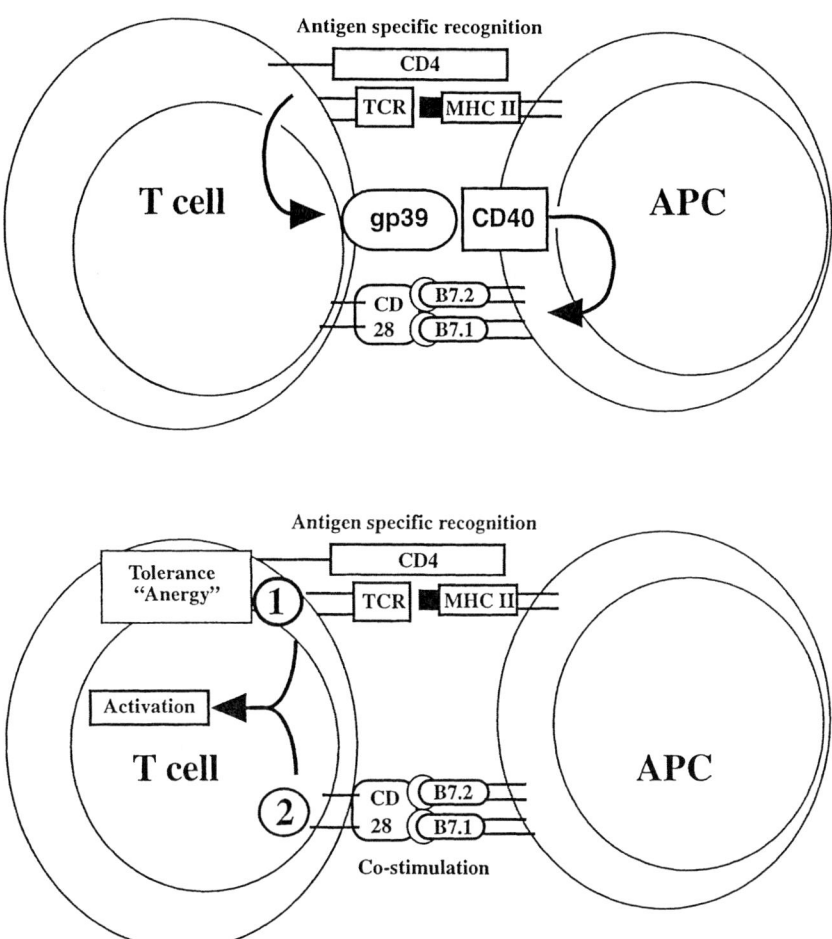

Figure 1. Regulation of T-cell activation by CD40 signaling. (Top panel) APC maturation is induced by CD40 signaling: Interaction of the TCR with Ag-MHC complex on the APC induces the expression of gp39 on the responding T-cell. (Bottom panel) T cell responses are governed by the availability of antigen-specific and co-stimulatory signals: Signal 1 only=tolerance, Signal 1+2=T cell activation: Expression of gp39 results in the engagement of CD40 on the cognate APC cell causing the upregulation of B7-1 and B7-2. As a consequence of increased expression of B7-1 and B7-2, the APC reciprocally trigger the T-cell *via* CD28 (2).

engagement can induce APC maturation. Once mature, APC then can more effectively stimulate T-cell proliferation. This is due to the upregulation of a host of co-stimulatory molecules (B7-1, B7-2, CD44] and the secretion of cytokines (IL-12) that can control the course of T-cell differentiation. In the absence of CD40 signaling, it appears that the APC compartment may not fully acquire the capacity to fully drive fulminant T-cell expansion.

References

1. Gordon, J., Millsum, M.J., Guy, G.R. and Ledbetter, J.A. (1987) Synergistic interaction between interleukin 4 and anti-Bp50 (CDw40) revealed in a novel B-cell restimulation assay. *Eur. J. Immunol.* 17: 1535.
2. Clark, E.A. and Ledbetter, J.A. (1986) Activation of human B-cells mediated through two distinct cell surface differentiation antigens, Bp35 and Bp 50. *Proc. Natl. Acad. Sci. USA* 83: 4494.
3. Stamenkovic, I., Clark, E.A. and Seed, B. (1989) A B-lymphocyte activation molecule related to the nerve growth factor receptor and induced by cytokines in carcinomas. *EMBO J.* 8: 1403.
4. Hollenbaugh, D., Grosmaire, L., Kullas, C.D., Chalupny, N.J., Noelle, R.J., Stamenkovic, I., Ledbetter, J.A. and Aruffo, A. (1992) The human T-cell antigen gp39, a member of the TNF gene family, is a ligand for the CD40 receptor: Expression of a soluble form of gp39 with B-cell co-stimulatory activity. *EMBO J.* 11: 4313.
5. Armitage, R.J., Fanslow, W.C., Strockbine, L., Sato, T.A., Clifford, K.N., Macduff, B.M., Anderson, D.M., Gimpel, S.D., Davis-Smith, T., Maliszewski, C.R., Clark, E.A., Smith, C.A., Grabstein, K.H., Cosman, D. and Spriggs, M.K. (1992) Molecular and biological characterization of a murine ligand for CD40. *Nature* 357: 80.
6. Valle, A., Zuber, C.E., Defrance, T., Djossou, O., De, R.M. and Banchereau, J. (1989) Activation of human B lymphocytes through CD40 and interleukin 4. *Eur. J. Immunol.* 19: 1463.
7. Gordon, J., Millsum, M.J., Flores, R.L. and Gillis, S. (1989) Regulation of resting and cycling human B lymphocytes *via* surface molecules interleukin-4, CD23 and CD40. *Immunology* 68: 526.
8. Jabara, H.H., Fu, S.M., Geha, R.S. and Vercelli D. (1990) CD40 and IgE: synergism between anti-CD40 monoclonal antibody and interleukin 4 in the induction of IgE synthesis by highly purified human B-cells. *J. Exp. Med.* 172: 1861.
9. Banchereau, J. and Rousset, F. (1991) Growing human B lymphocytes in the CD40 system. *Nature* 353: 678.
10. Armitage, R.J., Sato, T.A., Macduff, B.M., Clifford, K.N., Alpert, A.R., Smith, C.A. and Fanslow, W.C. (1992) Identification of a source of biologically active CD40 ligand. *Eur. J. Immunol.* 22: 2071.
11. Van den Eertwegh, A.J.M., Noelle, R.J., Roy, M., Shepherd, D.M., Aruffo, A., Ledbetter, J.A., Boersma, W.J.A. and Claassen E. (1993) *In vivo* CD40-gp39 interactions are essential for thymus-dependent immunity. I.CD40-gp39 interactions are essential for thymus dependent humoral immunity and identify sites of cognate interactions *in vivo*. *J. Exp. Med.* 178: 1555.
12. Noelle, R.J., Ledbetter, J.A. and Aruffo, A. (1992) CD40 and its ligand an essential ligand-receptor pair for thymus-dependent B-cell activation. *Immunol. Tod.* 13: 431.
13. Foy, T. Aruffo,, A., Bajorath, J., Buhlmann, J.E. and Noelle, R.J. (1996) Immune regulation by CD40 and its ligand gp39. *Ann. Rev. Immunol.* 14: 591.
14. Xu, J., Foy, T.M., Laman, J.D., Dunn, J.J., Waldschmidt, T.J., Elsemore, J., Noelle, R.J. and Flavell, R.A. (1994) Mice deficient for the CD40 ligand. *Immunity* 1: 423.
15. Renshaw, B.R., Fanslow, W., Armitage, R.J., Campbell, K.A., Liggitt, D., Wright, B., Davison, B.L. and Maliszewski, C.R. (1994) Humoral immune responses in CD40 ligand-deficient mice. *J. Exp. Med.* 180: 1889.
16. Kawabe, T., Naka, T., Yoshida, K., Tanaka, T., Fujiwara, H., Suematsu, S., Yoshida, N., Kishimoto, T. and Kikutani, H. (1994) The immune responses in CD40-deficient mice: impaired immunoglobulin class switching and germinal center formation. *Immunity* 1: 167.
17. Foy, T.M., Aruffo, A., Ledbetter, J.A. and Noelle, R.J. (1993) *In vivo* CD40-gp39 interactions are essential for thymus-dependent immunity. II. Prolonged *in vivo* suppression of primary and secondary humoral immune responses by an antibody targeted to the CD40 ligand gp39. *J. Exp. Med.* 178: 1567.
18. Foy, T.M., Laman, J.D., Ledbetter, J.A., Aruffo, A., Claassen, E. and Noelle, R.J. (1994) gp39-CD40 interactions are essential for germinal center formation and the development of B-cell memory. *J. Exp. Med.* 180: 157.
19. Gray, D., Dullforce, P. and Jainandunsing, S. (1994) Memory B-cell development but not germinal center formation is impaired by *in vivo* blockade of CD40-CD40-ligand interaction. *J. Exp. Med.* 184: 2399–2404.
20. Eynon, E.E. and Parker , D.(1992) Small B-cells as antigen-presenting cells in the induction of tolerance to soluble protein antigens. *J. Exp. Med.* 175: 131.
21. Harding, F.A. and Allison, J.P. (1993) CD28- B7 interactions allow the induction of CD8[+] cytotoxic T lymphocytes in the abscence of exogenous help. *J. Exp. Med.* 177: 1791.
22. Buhlmann, J.E., Foy, T.M., Aruffo, A., Crassi, K.M., Ledbetter, J.A., Green, W.R., Xu, J.C., Shultz, L.D., Roopesian, D., Flavell, R.A., Fast, L., Noelle, R.J. and Durie, F.H. (1995) In the absence of a CD40 Signal, B Cells Are Tolerogenic. *Immunity* 2: 645.
23. Parker, D.C., Greiner, D.L., Phillips, N.E., Appel, M.C., Steele, A.W., Durie, F.H., Noelle, R.J., Mordes, J.P. and Rossini, A.A. (1995) Survival of mouse pancreatic islet allografts in recipients treated with allogeneic small lymphocytes and antibody to CD40 ligand. *Proc. Natl. Acad. Sci.* 92: 9560.
24. Durie, F.H., Aruffo, A., Ledbetter, J.A., Crassi, K.M. Green, W.R. and Noelle, R.J. (1994) Antibody to the ligand of CD40, gp39, blocks the occurrence of the acute and chronic forms of graft- *versus*- host disease. *J. Clin. Invest.* 94: 1333.
25. Grewal, I.S., Xu, J. and Flavell, R.A. (1995) Impairment of antigen-specific T-cell priming in mice lacking CD40 ligand. *Nature* 378: 617.

AAS 49
Therapeutic Strategies for Modulating the Inflammatory Diseases
© 1998 Birkhäuser Verlag Basel/Switzerland

A role for inflammatory cytokines in the productive activation of antigen-specific CD4+ T-cells

K.A. Pape and M.K. Jenkins

Department of Microbiology and the Center for Immunology, University of Minnesota Medical School, 420 Delaware Street S.E., Minneapolis, MN 55455, USA

Summary. The mechanisms of action of immunological adjuvants were studied using a system in which the behavior of adoptively transferred CD4+ T-cell receptor transgenic T-cells could be directly monitored following antigen administration. These studies revealed that adjuvant-induced inflammatory cytokines promote immunity by enhancing the clonal expansion, persistence and differentiation of antigen-activated CD4+ T-cells.

Introduction

The immune system must walk a fine line between immunity and self-reactivity. CD4+ T-cells, each with a unique antigen receptor (TCR), are produced and selected in the thymus such that the emerging population of cells is capable of recognizing a multitude of antigenic peptides presented by the host's major histocompatibility complex (MHC) class II molecules. Because the process of TCR generation involves the random rearrangement of gene segments, it is unavoidable that T-cells specific for self peptide/class II MHC complexes will also be produced. One way the immune system deals with this situation is by subjecting the T-cells to a selection process in the thymus before the T-cells seed the secondary lymphoid organs. This process results in the clonal deletion of T-cells that recognize self peptide/class II MHC complexes on thymic antigen presenting cells (APCs) [1]. However, T-cells specific for self peptide/class II MHC complexes derived from developmentally regulated or tissue-specific proteins, which are not expressed in the thymus during maturation, will escape deletion and seed the periphery. Therefore, the immune system must have mechanisms to silence the function of these potentially autoreactive T-cells, and at the same time allow the function of T-cells specific for harmful antigens, such as those presented during microbial infection or trauma.

Early insights into this process came from studies on immunological adjuvants. In the early 1960's, experiments by David Dresser demonstrated that soluble foreign proteins were incapable of eliciting antibody production unless administered together with an adjuvant [2, 3]. Subsequent work showed that the injection of soluble antigen not only failed to induce an immune response [2], but actually induced a state of antigen-specific T-cell tolerance [4, 5]. Thus, although recognition of foreign antigen alone was sufficient for the induction of T-cell tolerance, additional signals, normally stimulated by bacterial molecules and mimicked by adjuvants, were required for T-cells to be productively activated. Decades later, and in spite of a myriad of experiments detailing the *in vitro* activation requirements of T-cells, the precise nature of the signals that adjuvants provide, and that may serve as "red flags" by which harmful agents are sensed, are not known. This has, in part, been due to a lack of methods to physically track the fate of antigen-specific lymphocytes in an intact organism. Recent technologies, such as the use of superantigens, that activate all T-cells that carry a particular TCR Vβ chain, and transgenic mice that express TCRs of known antigen specificity, allow for the tracking of antigen-stimulated T-cells with antibodies to particular Vβ chains or to the clonotypic TCR. The application of these new tools, in concert with our knowledge of *in vitro* CD4+ lymphocyte activation, is revealing new information on the adjuvant-induced *in vivo* signals that are required for the generation of functional helper T-cells.

Requirements for CD4+ T-cell activation and differentiation

In order to assess the points at which adjuvants may act to enhance T-cell immunity, it is useful to consider what is known about the activation requirements of CD4+ T-cells. Extensive *in vitro* studies have revealed that resting T-cells require signals through the TCR, as well as signals delivered through costimulatory molecules, to produce lymphokines and proliferate maximally [6]. The most well-characterized costimulatory system involves the CD28 molecule, which is constitutively expressed on T-cells, and the ligands, B7-1 and B7-2, which are expressed on activated bone-marrow derived APC [7]. Infusion of antibodies specific for B7-1 and B7-2, or a fusion protein that binds B7-1 and B7-2 (CTLA-4-Ig) inhibit T-cell clonal expansion following antigen priming [8, 9]. T-cell priming is also compromised in CD28-deficient mice [10], although not completely, potentially due to compensation by other costimulatory molecules. The critical role of CD28/B7-mediated costimulation is further indicated by the recent finding that the failure of T-cell priming in CD40 ligand (CD40L)-deficient mice may be an indirect effect of a lack of B7 induction on CD40+ APC [11–13].

Naïve T-cells, that receive appropriate signals through the TCR and costimulatory molecules, produce mainly IL-2, which acts as an autocrine growth factor for proliferation and clonal expansion [14]. Once activated, CD4+ T-cells then have the capacity to differentiate into cells that regulate different arms of the immune system. CD4+ T-cells of the Th1 type produce IL-2, IFN-γ and TNF-α, which promote B-cell switching to IgG2a and facilitate cell-mediated immune responses. Cells of the Th2 phenotype produce IL-4, IL-5 and IL-10, which promote B-cell switching to IgG1 and IgE, and favor humoral immune responses. It is thought that cytokines produced by cells of the innate immune system direct the development of naïve, antigen-stimulated CD4$^+$ T-cells into one of these T-helper subsets [15]. *In vitro* studies, using naïve TCR transgenic T-cells, have demonstrated that IL-12 plays a critical role in Th1 cell generation and is able to antagonize the function of IL-4, which is the major promoter of Th2 cell generation [16]. Furthermore, Th1 cells do not develop in IL-12-deficient mice [17], whereas Th2 cells do not develop in IL-4-deficient mice [18].

The effects of adjuvants

Many substances, including aluminum compounds, lipoidal compounds (Freund's adjuvant), and bacterial components (lipopolysaccharide (LPS), muramyl dipeptide) have been shown to have adjuvant activity [19]. Although adjuvants are thought to mimic an invading pathogenic microorganism by providing a prolonged source of antigen and by stimulating inflammation, the molecules responsible for adjuvant action have not been identified. Despite the fact that adjuvant components have been shown to induce cytokine production and surface expression of B7 and adhesion molecules on APCs *in vitro*, it has not been possible to assess the role these changes play in the priming of antigen-specific T-cells *in vivo*. To address this issue, our laboratory has developed a system where a small population of CD4$^+$ TCR transgenic T-cells, specific for ovalbumin, are adoptively transferred into normal syngeneic recipients, and tracked *in vivo* with an anti-clonotypic antibody specific for the transgenic TCR. This system approximates the physiological situation, where a small population of antigen-specific T-cells exist in a milieu of T-cells with different specificities.

We have used this system to monitor the behavior of antigen-specific T-cells following antigen injection in the presence or absence of adjuvant [20, 21]. When soluble antigen was injected along with an adjuvant (LPS or Freund's adjuvant), the antigen-specific T-cells expanded in a B7-dependent manner in the T-cell-rich paracortex of draining lymph nodes, persisted at elevated levels for many days and migrated into B-cell-rich follicles [20]. The transferred mice primed this way produced high levels of antigen-specific IgG1 and IgG2a [20] and developed a delayed-type hypersensitivity reaction when rechallenged with antigen (K.A. Pape and M.K. Jenkins, unpublished observation), suggesting that immunity was induced. A different profile was observed following injection of soluble antigen without adjuvant. Although transient B7-dependent expansion of the antigen-specific T-cells occurred, most of the T-cells did not persist in the lymphoid tissues or enter follicles, the mice made only low to undetectable levels of antigen-specific antibody [20], and antigenic rechallenge did not result in a delayed-type hypersensitivity reaction (K.A. Pape and M.K. Jenkins, unpublished observation). Transient activation and deletion of specific T-cells has also been described following injection of superantigens [21, 22] or class I-restricted peptides [22]. Thus, while injection of soluble foreign antigen alone causes the activation and transient B7-dependent clonal expansion of antigen-specific T-cells, this does not result in the generation of T-cells with helper function.

What then is missing in the T-cell response when antigen is injected alone and is present when antigen is injected with adjuvant? One possibility is inflammation. All adjuvants are thought to induce some inflammation, and LPS is particularly potent in this regard [23]. Using the adoptive transfer method described above, we tested this idea by determining whether the adjuvant effects of LPS could be substituted by inflammatory cytokines. Administration of either TNF-α or IL-1 enhanced the expansion and persistence of antigen-stimulated T-cells. Both TNF-α and IL-1 were also sufficient to induce the migration of antigen-activated T-cells into B-cell follicles and promote the production of antigen-specific IgG1. The interaction of antigen-specific T-cells with B-cells in follicles is thought to be critical for the formation of germinal centers [24]. Our results, together with recent findings that germinal center formation and antibody production is absent in TNF-receptor-deficient mice and TNF-α-deficient mice [25], are consistent with this idea. Furthermore, our results provide a physical basis for previous findings that IL-1 potentiates T-cell-dependent antibody responses and abrogates the induction of tolerance by soluble antigen [26–28].

Although TNF-α and IL-1 could account for the effects of LPS on the accumulation and migration of antigen-stimulated T-cells, they were not able to mimic the effects of LPS on the production of antigen-specific IgG2a. This function could be attributed to IL-12, since injection of exogenous IL-12 promoted the ability of the expanded population of antigen-specific T-cells to secrete IFN-γ in response to antigen, and resulted in the production of antigen-specific IgG2a. Thus, both TNF-α (or the IL-1 that it induces) and IL-12 were required to completely mimic the adjuvant effects of LPS.

In summary, *in vivo* systems that allow for the physical tracking of antigen-specific T-cells have revealed that T-cell activation and clonal expansion does not necessarily result in the generation of functional helper T-cells. Signals in addition to those delivered by the TCR and CD28 pathways, such as those provided by inflammatory cytokines, are also involved.

A model of *in vivo* T-cell activation

A model that takes into account the role of adjuvant-induced inflammation is shown in Figure 1. When soluble antigen enters peripheral lymphoid tissue in the absence of inflammation, it will be taken up by resident class II MHC+ APCs, processed and expressed as antigenic peptide/class II

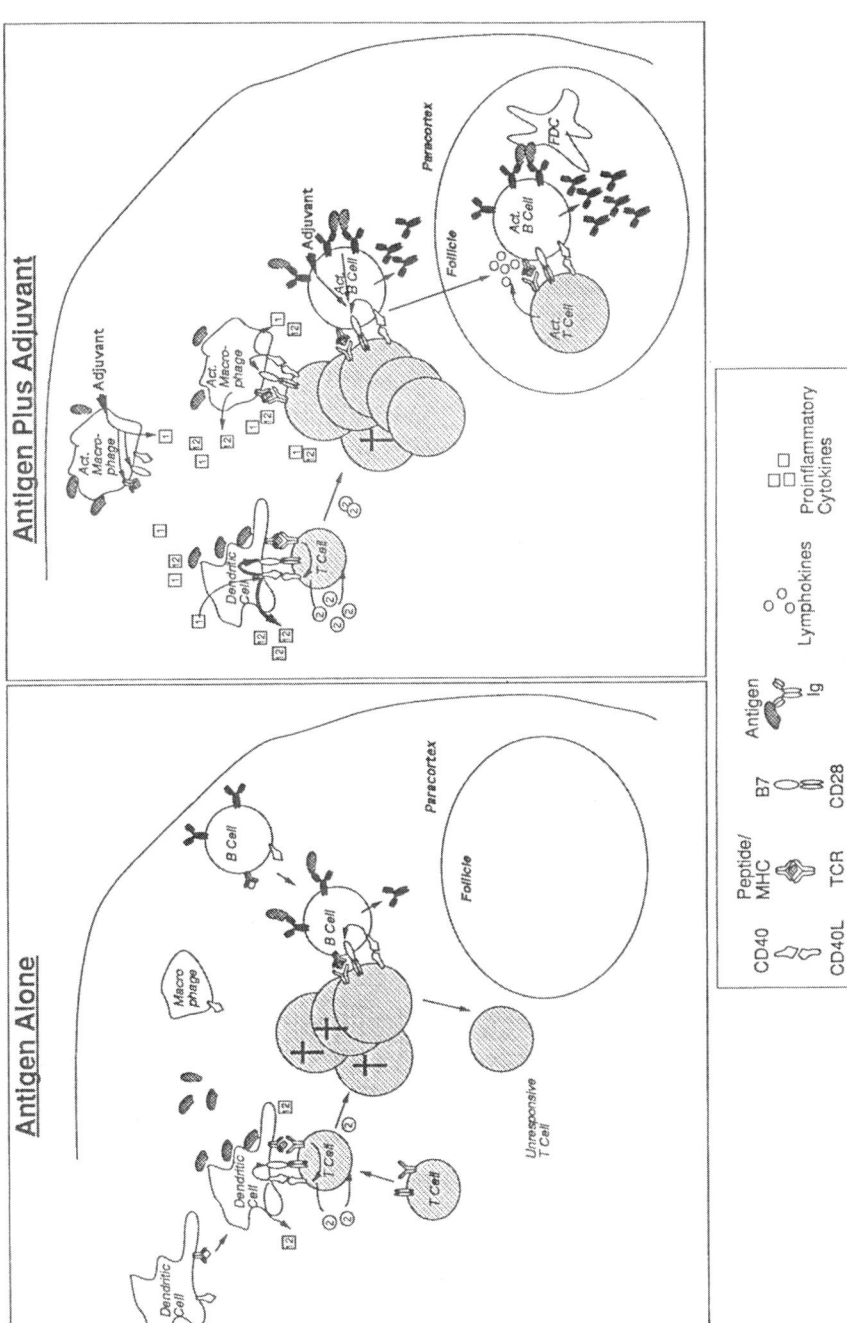

Figure 1. Activation of antigen-stimulated CD4⁺ T-cells in the presence or absence of adjuvant.

MHC complexes to naïve T-cells in T-cell-rich regions (e.g. the paracortex of lymph nodes, and the periarterial lymphoid sheath of the spleen). Dendritic cells are likely to be responsible for the majority of this antigen-presentation since they are the most abundant APC in the T-cell-rich regions, and form a reticular network that encompasses the T-cells. The dendritic cells that are present in secondary lymphoid tissues express B7-2 molecules *in situ*, although this level of expression is probably low and can be greatly increased when dendritic cells become activated. Steinman and colleagues have shown that splenic dendritic cells express high levels of class II MHC and adhesion molecules [29], and when pulsed with antigen *in vivo* are uniquely capable of stimulating T-cells *in vitro* [30]. Recognition of peptide/MHC complexes on dendritic cells would cause the responding T-cells to express CD40L, which would then bind to CD40 on the dendritic cell stimulating it to express more B7 and adhesion molecules, and to begin producing IL-12. The interacting T-cells would then be stimulated through the TCR and CD28, make IL-2, and begin to proliferate. However, in this model the T-cells rapidly decline in the absence of inflammation either because they die or migrate out of lymphoid tissue. They do not gain the ability to enter B-cell follicles or provide sufficient help for B-cell antibody production, and are left unresponsive to subsequent challenge with antigen.

The fate of antigen-stimulated T-cells is altered when adjuvant or pathogen-induced inflammation is present during antigen presentation. The production of inflammatory cytokines by macrophages at the site of injection or in the lymphoid tissue is likely to enhance the function of other APCs. A recent study demonstrated that T-cells specific for peptides derived from rat immunoglobulin became tolerant following injection of a rat antibody specific for dendritic cells, but were primed when the antibody was injected with IL-1 [31]. These results lead to the surprising suggestion that lymphoid dendritic cells are tolerogenic unless activated by an inflammatory stimulus. IL-1 amplifies the *in vitro* accessory cell function of dendritic cells by inducing more efficient clustering of dendritic cells with T-cells [32], and both TNF and IL-1 have been shown to increase the expression of CD40 on dendritic cells [33]. Thus, dendritic cells stimulated by CD40L expressing T-cells *in vivo* in the presence of inflammation would be expected to express enhanced levels of costimulatory molecules and adhesion molecules, and secrete increased amounts of IL-12 compared to unactivated dendritic cells.

Adjuvant or pathogen-induced activation of macrophage and B-cells could also result in enhanced ability of these APC to undergo productive interactions with T-cells. For example, LPS induces B7 molecules on resting B-cells *in vitro* [34]. There is some controversy, however, about whether activated B-cells are capable of priming naïve T-cells. Studies using antibodies to B-cell surface molecules have shown that while non-activating antibodies are tolerogenic for T-cells, activating antibodies induce a T-cell response, possibly due to their ability to increase the costimulatory function of B-cells [35–37]. However, Fuchs and Matzinger found that injection of both resting and activated male B-cells can induce tolerance in T-cells specific for the H-Y minor histocompatibility antigen [38]. In addition, Parker et al. found that although coexpression of B7 on human μ-chain-expressing B-cells could abrogate immunological tolerance to human μ-chain, it was not sufficient to induce an immune response [39]. Thus, interaction of naïve T-cells with activated B-cells does not always result in a productive T-cell response. It may be critical for naïve T-cells to first interact with inflammation-activated dendritic cells before becoming capable of engaging in productive interactions with other APC types that could serve to amplify the response. This scenario is consistent with findings that T-cell priming occurs in B-cell-deficient mice [40], but is often not as robust as T-cell priming in normal mice [41].

The precise mechanism whereby inflammatory cytokines promote the accumulation and retention of antigen-stimulated T-cells in lymph nodes is unknown. As stated above, inflammatory cytokines may increase the costimulatory activities of APCs such that interacting T-cells would be stimulated to produce more IL-2 and proliferate more extensively. Alternatively, inflammation may alter the efflux rate of antigen-stimulated T-cells such that they are retained in lymphoid tissue. Finally, adjuvant-or pathogen-induced inflammatory cytokines may prevent antigen-stimulated T-cells from dying as suggested by Vella et al. [42]. Future studies on the cell cycle status and survival protein expression pattern of antigen-stimulated T-cells will be required to resolve these possibilities.

In contrast, it is clear how adjuvants could affect the differentiation of antigen-stimulated T-cells. In situations where the adjuvant or pathogen induces a large amount of IL-12 production from the innate immune system cells, the expanding CD4$^+$ T-cell population would be induced to differentiate along the Th1 pathway, and result in IFN-γ-secreting T-cells that promote the production of antigen-specific IgG2a. If the adjuvant or infecting pathogen produces an IL-4-rich environment, then the CD4$^+$ T-cell population would differentiate along the Th2 pathway, resulting in IL-4 secreting T-cells that promote the production of antigen-specific IgG1 and IgE.

While immunologists have only recently started to understand the ways in which inflammatory cytokines signal the adaptive immune system, pathogenic organisms have been developing strategies to evade these signals for millions of years. Poxs viruses and some herpes viruses express receptors for IL-1, TNF and IFN-γ, which upon secretion from infected cells can sequester the cytokines and prevent them from binding to their natural receptors. Some strains of virus also express proteins which block processing of IL-1β to its mature secreted form. The Epstein-Barr virus and Equine herpes virus type 2 produce homologues of IL-10, which can inhibit IL-12 production from macrophages [43, 44]. By inhibiting inflammation microbes benefit not only because non-specific immune mechanisms are impaired, but also because CD4$^+$ T-cells, and all of the effector responses that depend on them, will be primed less efficiently.

References

1. Sprent, J. and Webb, S.R. (1995) Intrathymic and extrathymic clonal deletion of T-cells. *Curr. Opin. Immunol.* 7: 196–205.
2. Dresser D.W. (1961) Effectiveness of lipid and lipidophilic substances as adjuvants. *Nature* 191: 1169–1171.
3. Freund, J., Casals, J. and Hosmer, E.P. (1937) Sensitization and antibody formation after injection of tubercle bacilli and paraffin oil. *Proc. Soc. Exp. Biol. Med.* 37: 509–513.
4. Parks, D.E. and Weigle, W.O. (1980) Current perspectives on the cellular mechanisms of immunologic tolerance. *Clin. Exp. Immunol.* 39: 257–262.
5. Chiller, J.M., Habicht, G.S. and Weigle, W.O. (1961) Kinetic differences in unresponsiveness of thymus and bone marrow cells. *Science* 171: 813–815.
6. Mueller, D.L., Jenkins, M.K. and Schwartz, R.H. (1989) Clonal expansion *versus* functional clonal inactivation: a costimulatory signaling pathway determines the outcome of T-cell antigen receptor occupancy. *Ann. Rev. Immunol.* 7: 445–490.
7. Lenschow, D.J., Walunas, T.L. and Bluestone, J.A. (1996) CD28/B7 system of T-cell costimulation. *Ann. Rev. Immunol.* 14: 233–258.
8. Linsley, P.S., Wallace, P.M., Johnson, J., Gibson, M.G., Greene, J.L., Ledbetter, J.A., Singh, C. and Tepper, M.A. (1992) Immunosuppression *in vivo* by a soluble form of the CTLA-4 T-cell activation molecule. *Science* 257: 792–795.
9. Kearney, E.R., Walunas, T.L., Karr, R.W., Morton, P.A., Loh, D.Y., Bluestone, J.A. and Jenkins, M.K. (1995) Antigen-dependent clonal expansion of a trace population of antigen-specific CD4$^+$ T-cells *in vivo* is dependent on CD28 costimulation and inhibited by CTLA-4. *J. Immunol.* 155: 1032–1036.
10. Green, J.G., Noel, P., Sperling, A.I., Walunas, T.L., Gray, G.S., Bluestone, J.A. and Thompson, C.B. (1994) Absence of B7-dependent responses in CD28-deficient mice. *Immunity* 1: 501–508.
11. Grewal, I.S., Xu, J. and Flavell R.A. (1995) Impairment of antigen-specific T-cell priming in mice lacking CD40 ligand. *Nature* 378: 617–620.
12. Grewal, I.S., Foellmer, H.G., Grewal, K.D., Xu, J., Hardardottir, F., Baron JL, Jr. C.A.J. and Flavell RA (1996) Requirement for CD40 ligand in costimulation induction, T-cell activation, and experimental allergic encephalomyelitis. *Science* 273: 1864–1867.
13. Yang, Y. and Wilson, J.M. (1996) CD40 ligand-dependent T-cell activation: Requirement of B7-CD28 signaling through CD40. *Science* 273: 1862–1864.
14. Swain, S.L., Weinberg, A.D. and English, M. (1990) CD4$^+$ T-cell subsets: lymphokine secretion of memory cells and of effector cells that develop from precursors. *J. Immunol.* 144: 1788–1799.
15. Paul, W.E. and Seder, R.A. (1994) Lymphocyte responses and cytokines. *Cell* 76: 241–251.
16. Trinchieri G. (1995) IL-12: A proinflammatory cytokine with immunoregulatory functions that bridge innate resistance and antigen-specific adaptive immunity. *Ann. Rev. Immunol.* 13: 251–276.
17. Magram, J., Connaughton, S.E., Warrier, R.R., Carvajal, D.M., Wu CY, Ferreante, J., Stewart, C., Sermiento, U., Faherty DA and Gately MK (1996) IL-12-deficient mice are defective in IFN-gamma production and type 1 cytokine responses. *Immunity* 4: 471–481.
18. Kuhn, R., Rajewsky, K. and Muller, W. (1991) Generation and analysis of IL-4 deficient mice. *Science* 254: 707–710.
19. Warren, H.S., Vogel, F.R. and Chedid, L.A. (1986) Current status of immunological adjuvants. *Ann. Rev. Immunol.* 4: 369–388.
20. Pape, K.A., Mondino, A., Khoruts, A. and Jenkins, M.K. (1996) Inflammatory cytokines and prolonged antigen-presentation enhance the *in vivo* persistence and differentiation of antigen-activated CD4$^+$ T-cells. *J. Immunol.* 159: 591–598.
21. Kearney, E.R., Pape, K.A., Loh, D.Y. and Jenkins, M.K. (1994) Visualization of peptide-specific T-cell immunity and peripheral tolerance induction *in vivo*. *Immunity* 1: 327–339.
22. Kyburz, D., Aichele, P., Speiser, D.E., Hengartner, H., Zinkernagel, R.M. and Pircher, H. (1993) T-cell immunity after a viral infection *versus* T-cell tolerance induced by soluble viral peptides. *Eur. J. Immunol.* 23: 1956–1962.
23. Brouckaert, P., Libert ,C., Everaerdt, B., Takahashi, N,. Cauwels, A. and Fiers, W. (1993) Tumor necrosis factor, its receptors and the connection with interleukin 1 and interleukin 6. *Immunobiol.* 187: 317–329.
24. Kelso, G. (1994) B-cell diversification and differentiation in the periphery. *J. Exp. Med.* 180: 5–6.
25. Liu, Y.-J. and Banchereau, J. (1996) Mutant mice without B lymphocyte follicles. *J. Exp. Med.* 184: 1207–1211.
26. Weigle, W.O., Scheuer, W.V., Hobbs, M.V., Morgan, E.L. and Parks, D.E. (1987) Modulation of the induction and circumvention of immunological tolerance to human g-globulin by interleukin 1. *J. Immunol.* 138: 2069–2074.
27. Reed, S.G., Pihl, D.L., Conlon, P.J. and Grabstein, K.H. (1989) Role of T-cells in the augmentation of specific antibody production by recombinant human IL-1α. *J. Immunol.* 142: 3129–3133.
28. Nohria, A. and Rubin, R. (1994) Cytokines as potential vaccine adjuvants. *Biotherapy* 7: 261–269.

29. Steinman R.M. (1991) The dendritic cell system and its role in immunogenicity. *Ann. Rev. Immunol.* 9: 271–296.
30. Crowley, M., Inaba, K. and Steinman, R.M. (1990) Dendritic cells are the principal cells in mouse spleen bearing immunogenic fragments of foreign proteins. *J. Exp. Med.* 172: 383–386.
31. Finkelman, F.D., Lees, A., Birnbaum, R., Gause, W.C. and Morris, S.C. (1996) Dendritic cells can present antigen *in vivo* in a tolerogenic or immunogenic fashion. *J. Immunol.* 157: 1406–1414.
32. Koide, S.L., Inaba, K. and Steinman, R. (1987) Interleukin 1 enhances T-dependent immune responses by amplifying the function of dendritic cells. *J. Exp. Med.* 165: 515–530.
33. McLellan, A.D., Sorg, R.V., Williams, L.A. and Hart, D.N.J. (1996) Human dendritic cells activate T lymphocytes *via* a CD40:CD40 ligand-dependent pathway. *Eur. J. Immunol.* 26: 1204–1210.
34. Liu, Y. and Janeway, C.A. Jr. (1991) Microbial induction of co-stimulatory activity for CD4 T-cell growth. *Int. Immunol.* 3: 323–332.
35. Morris, S.C., Lees, A. and Finkelman, F.D. (1994) *In vivo* activation of naïve T-cells by antigen-presenting B-cells. *J. Immunol.* 152: 3777–3785.
36. Morris, S.C., Lees, A., Holmes, J.M., Jeffries, R.D.A. and Finkelman, F.D. (1994) Induction of B-cell and T-cell tolerance *in vivo* by anti-CD32 mAb. *J. Immunol.* 152: 3726–3776.
37. Eynon, E.E. and Parker, D.C. (1993) Parameters of tolerance induction by antigen targeted to B lymphocytes. *J. Immunol.* 151: 2958–2964.
38. Fuchs, E.J. and Matzinger, P. (1992) B-cell turn off virgin but not memory T-cells. *Science* 258: 1156–1159.
39. Yuschenkoff ,V.N., Sethna, M.P., Freeman, G.J. and Parker, D.C. (1996) Coexpression of B7-1 and antigen blocks tolerance induction to antigen presented by resting B-cells. *J. Immunol.* 157: 1987–1995.
40. Epstein, M.M., Rosa, F.D., Jankovic, D., Sher, A. and Matzinger, P. (1995) Successful T-cell priming in B-cell-deficient mice. *J. Exp. Med.* 182: 915–922.
41. Vella, A.T., Scherer, M.T., Shultz, L., Kappler, J.W. and Marrack, P. (1996) B-cells are not essential for peripheral T-cell tolerance induction. *Proc. Natl. Acad. Sci. USA* 93: 951–955.
42. Vella, A.T., McCormack, J.E., Linsley, P.S., Kappler, J.W. and Marrack, P. (1995) Lipolysaccharide interferes with the induction of peripheral T-cell death. *Immunity* 2: 261–270.
43. Smith, G.L. (1994) Virus strategies for evasion of the host response to infection. *Trends Microbiol.* 2: 81–88.
44. Marrack, P. and Kappler, J. (1994) Subversion of the immune system by pathogens. *Cell* 76: 323–332.

AAS 49
Therapeutic Strategies for Modulating the Inflammatory Diseases
© 1998 Birkhäuser Verlag Basel/Switzerland

The complexity of the B7-CD28/CTLA-4 costimulatory pathway

A.N. Schweitzer and A.H. Sharpe

Brigham and Women's Hospital and Harvard Medical School, Boston, MA, USA

Summary. There have been significant recent advances in our understanding of the role of the B7-CD28/CTLA-4 costimulatory pathway in T-cell activation and self-tolerance. Recent studies have begun to clarify how signaling through this pathway can influence cytokine production. The critical role for CTLA-4 in regulating T-cell activation and autoreactivity has been demonstrated, revealing a previously unsuspected means by which costimulation is involved in the maintenance and breakdown of self-tolerance. *In vivo* studies indicate the therapeutic potential of manipulating this important, but complex, immunoregulatory pathway.

Introduction

The concept of costimulation refers to the idea that lymphocytes need stimuli in addition to antigen to manifest their complete response profiles. For optimal activation, T-cells need to receive a first signal mediated by recognition of antigen/MHC complexes by TCR (T-cell receptor) in conjunction with a second "co-stimulatory signal". Importantly, because costimulation prevents induction of a state of anergy to subsequent activation in the responding T-cells [1], there is great interest in manipulating costimulatory pathways for therapeutic purposes. Inhibiting costimulatory signals may enable novel antigen-specific therapeutic approaches for controlling undesirable T-cell responses in autoimmune diseases, allergies and graft-*versus*-host disease, whereas enhancing costimulatory signals provides a means to augment T-cell responses to tumors and infectious agents. Several ligand-receptor pairs have been identified which promote T-cell proliferation upon CD3/TCR signaling [2]. However, a prominent role for interactions between B7 molecules B7-1 and B7-2 on the APC (antigen presenting cell), and CD28 on the T-cell, has emerged due to the unique capacity of B7-CD28 signaling to prevent the induction of anergy *in vitro* [3, 4]. Recently, it has become clear that the role of B7 molecules may be far more complex than one of simple costimulation, and that the concept of costimulation may, indeed, require modification. In this review we focus on recent studies which have investigated the role of B7-CD28 signals in regulating Th1 *versus* Th2 responses, and the recently discovered critical role of the second B7 ligand, CTLA-4, in negatively regulating T-cell activation and maintaining immunological homeostasis.

Receptors and ligands in the B7-CD28/CTLA-4 pathway

The potential complexity of the B7-CD28/CTLA-4 pathway is evident from the existence of at least two ligands, B7-1 (CD80) and B7-2 (CD86), and two receptors, CD28 and CTLA-4 [5]. B7-2 is constitutively expressed on dendritic cells, macrophages and T-cells, and expression is rapidly induced or enhanced on APCs and T-cells in response to numerous stimuli, whereas B7-1 appears more slowly and often at significantly lower levels [4, 5] The constitutive or early expression of B7-2 has led to the hypothesis that B7-2 may participate in initiating an immune response, thereby playing a pivotal role in the decision between T-cell activation and anergy, whereas B7-1, being expressed later, may serve to amplify or regulate an immune response. CD28 is constitutively expressed at the T-cell surface, whereas CTLA-4 is mainly found intracellularly, and cell surface expression is induced only upon activation [6]. While the role of CD28 in T-cell activation is well established [3–5], the critical role of CTLA-4 as a negative regulator of T-cell activation and autoimmunity has been illuminated during the past year [7, 8].

While mitogenic stimulation with LPS induces expression of both B7-1 and B7-2, induction of minimal or no detectable B7-1 expression has been associated with several stimuli related to antigen-specific responses, namely following antigen-specific activation of B-cells *in vivo* [9] and Ig-receptor mediated activation of B-cells *in vitro* [4]. Ligation of MHC molecules at the time of B-cell activation *via* CD40 can inhibit CD40-mediated induction of B7-1 expression [10]. Expression of B7-1 and B7-2 can also vary according to the chronicity of stimulation. For example, during the early stages of murine experimental autoimmune encephalomyelitis (EAE), a T-cell-mediated model of autoimmune disease, B7-2 is the predominant costimulatory molecule detected in the CNS, whereas B7-1 expression predominates at later stages of disease [11]. Cytokines and infectious agents can influence the expression of B7-1 and B7-2 in both a positive and a negative fashion [12].

Whether B7-1 and B7-2 are functionally distinct is controversial. Some investigators have reported differences in CD4$^+$ T-cell cytokine profiles in the presence of one *versus* the other [13–15] and distinct capacities to costimulate development of CD8$^+$ cytotoxic cells [16], while other investigators find no differences [17]. Our results suggest that differences in the level and/or kinetics of B7 expression may account for observed differences [18], as we will discuss below.

B7-1 and B7-2 have similar low affinities for CD28 and high affinities for CTLA-4, but they have distinct kinetics of binding to CD28 and CTLA-4, with B7-2 having faster dissociation kinetics [6]. The distinct affinities of B7 ligands for CD28 and CTLA-4 could potentially influence whether B7-CD28 or B7-CTLA-4 interactions predominate at distinct stages of an immune response. For example, when B7 ligands are expressed at low levels, these costimulators might preferentially engage the high-affinity inhibitory receptor, CTLA-4. In contrast, when the

B7 ligands are upregulated and expressed at high levels, such as upon encounter with immuno-genic antigens or adjuvants, the predominant interactions could be between CD28 and B7, leading to T-cell proliferation and differentiation. As CTLA-4 expression becomes upregulated following T-cell activation, the inhibitory B7-CTLA-4 interaction would once again predominate and T-cell activation would be terminated. Specific reagents which enable the testing of these hypotheses have become available only recently, and should enhance our understanding of the interactions among receptors and ligands in this pathway.

B7-CD28/CTLA-4 interactions and cytokine production

CD4+ T-cell effector function comprises two distinct phenotypes, the Th1 response characterized by production of IL-2, IFN-γ and TNF-ß and associated with inflammatory "cell-mediated" responses, and the Th2 response characterized by production of IL-4, IL-5 and IL-10 associated with the down-regulation of inflammation and with certain forms of humoral immunity [19] The physiological mechanisms of subset differentiation remain unclear. Factors which can influence subset differentiation in experimental systems include host genetic background, cytokine milieu at the time of T-cell priming, antigen dose and route of immunization (for review see [20]).

The influence of B7-CD28/CTLA-4 interactions upon cytokine production appears to depend upon both the activation state of the responding T-cell and the experimental system examined. Blockade of the B7-CD28/CTLA-4 pathway during primary T-cell stimulation can inhibit pro-duction of both IL-2 and IL-4 *in vitro* [21] and *in vivo* [22, 23]. In contrast, following pre-stimu-lation, or blockade of the B7-CD28/CTLA-4 pathway with CTLA-4Ig subsequent to antigen exposure, sensitivity of Th1- but not Th2-type responses to B7-CD28/CTLA-4 blockade is observed in a number of *in vitro* and *in vivo* systems [24–26]. B7-CD28/CTLA-4 blockade at the time of infection with *Leishmania major* skews the usual Th2 response of susceptible mice to-wards a curative Th1 response, while having no effect upon Th1 responses of resistant mice [27]. Immunization of CD28 deficient mice with KLH results in diminished levels of IL-4 production upon *in vitro* restimulation, but retained IFN–γ production [28], supporting an important role for signaling through CD28 in the induction of IL-4 production. However, *L. major* infection of CD28 deficient mice backcrossed onto either resistant or susceptible backgrounds proceeds as in wild type mice and wild type levels of Th1 and Th2 responses, respectively, can be measured *ex vivo* [28]. *In vitro* studies had previously shown that high concentrations of antigen were able to stimulate IL-2 production and proliferation by TCR transgenic T-cells from CD28 deficient mice. Nevertheless, CD28 signaling was necessary for induction of high levels of IL-2 production and sustained proliferation, and for upregulating the expression of the cell survival molecule Bcl-x

[29]. These results suggest that many factors, including the duration and magnitude of antigen exposure, may affect the extent to which the B7-CD28/CTLA-4 pathway is required for induction of cytokine synthesis.

A potential role for B7-1 *versus* B7-2 in influencing the cytokine profile of T-cells has been implicated in a number of *in vitro* and *in vivo* models of T-cell activation [13–15]. However, the observed influence differs according to the model: For example, anti-B7-1 antibodies depress and anti-B7-2 antibodies exacerbate peptide-induced, Th1-mediated EAE [14], consistent with studies showing that CHO cells transfected with B7-2 stimulate human T-cells to produce IL-4 [13]. In contrast, anti-B7-1 exacerbates and anti-B7-2 protects against Th1-mediated diabetes in NOD mice [15].

We have used APCs from mice lacking expression of either B7-1 or B7-2 to stimulate TCR transgenic T-cells and examine the cytokine profile following a second round of stimulation using wild type APCs [18]. Our results indicate that B7-mediated costimulation significantly contributes to both IFN-γ and IL-4 production especially when T-cells are primed under sub-optimal conditions, with a greater influence of B7-2 than B7-1. Our results suggest that B7 molecules may simply contribute to the strength of the primary response which in turn influences the cytokine profile upon restimulation. Production of IL-4 following a second round of stimulation was particularly sensitive to the strength of the primary response. Induction of IFN-γ and IL-2 production were also sensitive, but were still induced to some extent in the absence of measurable IL-4 when priming conditions were sub-optimal. We believe that the autocrine nature of Th2 response differentiation in response to IL-4 accounts for the particular sensitivity of secondary IL-4 production to priming conditions; less IL-4 production during priming would result in the differentiation of fewer Th2-like cells, whereas Th1 development would be more dependent on additional non-T-cell derived factors such as IL-12. The greater effect of B7-2 than B7-1 in our system appeared to reflect the predominance of B7-2 expression as compared with B7-1 expression at all time points examined.

Our studies examining the effect of stimulus strength upon the induction of cytokine production provide a basis for understanding the apparently contradictory results which have emerged concerning the relationship between B7-1, B7-2 and cytokine induction. The discrepancy between the outcome of anti-B7-2 treatment of murine diabetes and EAE may be explained as follows: EAE is induced using potent antigen and inflammatory stimuli (leading to IL-2, IFN-γ and IL-4 production), which may relate most closely to a high strength of stimulus in our *in vitro* studies [18]. During EAE, the expression of B7-1 and B7-2 varies according to the chronicity of stimulation; early in disease induction, B7-2 is the predominant costimulatory molecule detected in the CNS, whereas B7-1 predominates later [11]. Blockade of B7-2 from the time of disease induction onwards exacerbates disease [14], consistent with the idea that B7-2 is required for priming for Th2 development, and that IL-4 may be depressing the development of Th1 responses during induction of EAE. The reason why B7-2 blockade has this effect but anti-B7-1 does not is most likely because B7-2 is the principal costimulator early during immune response induction. B7-1 appears later, and anti-B7-1 suppressed disease (i.e. sustained Th1 activation) in this model. Cessation of anti-B7-1 treatment results in worsening of the B7-1-protected state [14], consistent with a predominant contribution of B7-1 to ongoing stimulation of IFN-γ production. In contrast, diabetes in the NOD mouse is a spontaneous disease which develops gradually, suggesting that the stimulus may be less intense. Under these conditions, IL-4 production may be minimal and IL-2 and IFN-γ production may be more sensitive to B7 blockade in parallel with our results. B7-2 expression appears to predominate both prior to and following pancreatic infiltration in the NOD mouse model of IDDM [30], which would explain the protective effects of anti-B7-2 treatment in this model [15]. The disease-exacerbating effects of anti-B7-1 treatment in NOD mice, however, lie beyond the scope of our present understanding of the pathway. It is possible that instead of blocking interactions with their receptors, anti-B7 mAbs could, under certain circumstances, have activating properties and lead to signaling into the T-cell or the APC *in vivo*. Indeed, recent *in vitro* studies suggest that anti-B7-1 not only can block costimulation *via* APCs, but also can signal into cells expressing B7 molecules [31, 32].

CTLA-4 as a negative regulator of T-cell activation and auto-reactivity

The first insight into a negative regulatory role for CTLA-4 came from studies using anti-CTLA-4 monoclonal antibodies [33–35]. Earlier studies had suggested that anti-CTLA-4 mAbs augmented proliferation of T-cells stimulated with anti-CD3 [6], but it is now thought that the mAbs were blocking an inhibitory interaction between B7 and CTLA-4 rather than transducing a positive signal [33–35]. In the absence of anti-CD28 mAb, anti-CTLA-4 mAb did not provide a costimulatory signal to purified T-cells activated with anti-CD3. Monovalent Fab fragments of anti-CTLA-4 mAb, which block CTLA-4-B7 interactions and presumably are unable to signal, augmented proliferation of purified T-cells activated with anti-CD3 and costimulated with anti-CD28, analogous to the effect of soluble anti-CTLA-4 mAbs. Conversely, under conditions of Fc crosslinking, anti-CTLA-4 mAb inhibited T-cell proliferation. *In vivo* studies using anti-CTLA-4 mAbs also support an inhibitory function for CTLA-4. Either intact anti-CTLA-4 mAb or Fab fragments increased the expansion of T-cells reactive with specific peptide antigen [36].

The phenotype of mice lacking CTLA-4 (CTLA-4 -/-) provided direct evidence for the critical physiological role for CTLA-4 in negatively regulating T-cell activation and autoreactivity [7, 8]. These mice rapidly developed a spontaneous lymphoproliferative disease with massive lymphocytic infiltrates and tissue destruction in many organs. Mice exhibited splenomegaly, lymphade-nopathy, and elevated serum immunoglobulin levels and died by 3–4 weeks of age. The peripheral T-cells from these mice were activated, proliferated spontaneously *in vitro*, and produced abundant cytokines. The lymphoproliferation in these mice could reflect a failure to delete potentially autoreactive cells in the thymus, a failure to terminate antigen-specific T-cell proliferative responses, or a failure of antigen-specific apoptosis of activated T lymphocytes. In fact, the thymic profile of CTLA-4 -/- mice was altered, with a marked reduction in the percentage of double positive CD4+CD8+ thymocytes, a relative increase in single positive CD3+CD4+ and CD3+CD8+ thymocytes, and an increase in double negative CD4−CD8− thymocytes, as compared to wild type mice. It remains to be determined whether this abnormal thymic phenotype truly reflects abnormal lymphocyte development, or whether infiltration of the thymus by single-positive cells from the periphery is occurring, consistent with a peripheral CTLA-4 regulatory mechanism. Nevertheless, the striking phenotype of the CTLA-4 -/- mouse demonstrates a critical role for CTLA-4 in regulating T-cell activation and maintaining immunologic homeostasis. Furthermore, it is clear that signaling through CD28 and CTLA-4 can have opposing effects, and that the outcome of an immune response involves a balance between CD28-mediated T-cell activation and CTLA-4-mediated down-regulation.

While the phenotype of the CTLA-4 -/- mouse provided the first formal proof that dysregulation of costimulation can result in activation of T-cells that mediate lethal tissue injury, the outcome contrasted with the original expectation that absence of costimulatory ligands and/or receptors would lead to tolerance. Indeed, it appears that the B7-CD28/CTLA-4 pathway plays an essential role in maintaining tolerance to self antigens and that negative signaling *via* CTLA-4 plays an active role in regulating autoreactive T-cells. A recent study examining immune responses of transgenic mice expressing soluble CTLA-4Ig supports this hypothesis [37]. CTLA-4Ig was found to prevent, rather than facilitate, tolerance induction in CD4+ T-cells, suggesting that signaling *via* a B7-dependent mechanism is needed to induce tolerance.

In addition to providing key insights into the function of CTLA-4, the CTLA-4 deficient mouse strain also represents a unique model of spontaneous, multi-organ T-cell-mediated tissue damage. Spontaneous models of autoimmunity can prove instructive in offering insights into the molecular and genetic basis of autoimmune diseases. It is of particular interest to compare the phenotype of CTLA-4 -/- mice with that of mice with mutations in *fas* (*lpr/lpr*) and *fas* ligand (*gld/gld*). The latter mice develop a spontaneous autoimmune lupus-like disease and have provided useful models for analyzing mechanisms of self-tolerance and autoimmunity [38] and demonstrated a critical role for *Fas-FasL*-mediated apoptosis in the deletion of self-reactive T-cells in the periphery. However, unlike the CTLA-4 deficient mice, *lpr/lpr* and *gld/gld* mice do not develop multi-organ T-cell-infiltrative disease. This implies that distinct mechanisms may be responsible for maintaining tolerance to disseminated and tissue-specific self antigens. Under-standing the mechanisms which govern self-tolerance to distinct autoantigens should facilitate development of rational therapeutic strategies for spontaneous autoimmune diseases.

The critical immunoregulatory function of CTLA-4 suggests that blockade of CTLA-4 signaling could be used to boost otherwise sub-optimal immune responses such as those directed against tumors. Administration of anti-CTLA-4 mAbs stimulated anti-tumor immunity in mice, resulting in striking tumor regression even in mice with established tumors, and in immunity to rechallenge with tumor [39]. It remains to be established whether this effect is, in fact, due to blockade of negative signaling though CTLA-4, or to direct stimulation of anti-tumor-specific T-cells. Administration of anti-CTLA-4 mAb to recipients of PLP 139–151-specific T-cells led to accelerated and more severe disease [40], consistent with the effect of anti-CTLA-4 mAb in boosting anti-tumor immunity. Together, these studies demonstrate the potential utility of mani-pulating CTLA-4 to enhance immune responses and potentially also to block activated T-cells mediating autoimmune responses.

Two possible mechanisms by which CTLA-4 exerts the observed negative regulatory function have been implicated. A role in terminating T-cell responses by inducing cell death was suggested by one study using an anti-CTLA-4 mAb which binds an epitope distinct from all other reported anti-CTLA-4 mAbs [41], and uniquely does not interfere with CTLA-4 binding to B7-1 or B7-2 [34]. This antibody induced cell death in human T-cells incubated with antigen. Two studies have evaluated the potential for CTLA-4 to regulate T-cell activation by interfering with events associ-ated with T-cell activation, such as gene expression, growth factor or survival factor production, or cell cycle progression. Studies using anti-CTLA-4 mAbs have indicated that CTLA-4 signaling may block CD28-dependent IL-2 production, IL-2R expression and cell cycle progression of activated T-cells, arresting cells in G0/G1.

Another recent study has provided the first insight into the nature of the intracellular signaling pathways by which CTLA-4 exerts its inhibitory effects [43]. The tyrosine kinases, FYN, LCK, and ZAP-70, and the RAS pathway are constitutively activated in CTLA-4 -/- T-cells. Therefore, a role for CTLA-4 in negatively regulating proximal signaling events after TCR activation has been inferred. These studies showed a specific association of CTLA-4 with the tyrosine phosphatase SYP (PTP1d) and suggest that CTLA-4 regulates CD28 mediated activation of tyrosine kinases through the tyrosine phosphatase, SYP. This exciting finding draws parallels between the roles of protein tyrosine phosphatases in negatively regulating B-cells, T-cells, and NK cells [44]. For example, the tyrosine phosphatase SHP (PTP1c) associates with the CD22 receptor and FcγRIIb in B-cells and SHP deficient (motheaten) mice exhibit hyperactivation of B-cell receptor signaling pathways.

Conclusion

Manipulation of the B7:CD28/CTLA-4 costimulatory pathway may enable a distinctive immuno-regulatory strategy for achieving transplantation tolerance, for controlling allergies and autoimmune diseases, and for inducing immunity to infectious agents and tumors. Methods interfering with signaling through this pathway would affect only those antigen-specific T-cells undergoing activation and not have global effects on immune responses. By blocking the crucial second signal at the time of antigen recognition, only those T-cells responding to antigen would be affected and rendered anergic to antigen. Costimulatory blockade may be particularly advantageous for therapy of autoimmune diseases, where the precise antigens eliciting autoimmune T-cell activation are uncertain. In contrast to therapies that interfere with TCR recognition, manipulation of costimulatory signals does not require identification of the antigen or of individual polymorphic MHC and TCR. Thus, manipulation of costimulatory signals may provide a broadly applicable therapeutic approach for manipulating T-cell activation, unlike the extremely specific therapeutic maneuvers that interfere with TCR-mediated signals and necessitate an individualized therapy for each patient.

Given the complexity of the B7-CD28/CTLA-4 pathway which has emerged recently, it is perhaps not surprising that ongoing studies involving blockade of this pathway have met with mixed success. CTLA-4Ig treatment can prevent graft rejection and lead to prolonged and even indefinite survival of pancreatic, cardiac, renal and bone marrow transplants [45, 46]. Manipulation of the B7-CD28/CTLA-4 costimulatory pathway also can prevent the initiation of an autoimmune responses, as well as suppress an ongoing autoimmune process (for review, see [47]). The effectiveness of CTLA-4Ig on established disease is particularly interesting, since most autoimmune diseases are diagnosed after initial responses to the autoantigens. Significantly, the profound inhibition of the clinical and histological manifestations of an autoimmune disease (e.g., EAE) continued after cessation of CTLA-4Ig treatment [48]. The mechanism by which CTLA-4Ig exerts protective effects is not yet clear. Certain CTLA-4Ig treatment protocols, however, exacerbated rather than ameliorated autoimmune disease. The timing of CTLA-4-Ig administration appears to be a critical factor in influencing the outcome of treatment [31]. These results may reflect the complex coordinated interactions among B7-1, B7-2, CD28 and CTLA-4, and suggest that there may be opposing effects upon the outcome of an immune response, depending upon whether positive or negative signaling capabilities of the pathway are disrupted. Furthermore, as discussed above, Th1 versus Th2 cytokine production can be influenced by B7-1 and B7-2 via the contribution of B7 costimulatory molecules to the strength of stimulus received by T-cells. Thus, disruption of B7-receptor interactions may affect cytokine balance, and result in either harmful inflammatory Th1 effects or beneficial protective Th2 responses *in vivo* depending upon the timing and amount of B7 and antigen present.

The critical negative immunoregulatory role of CTLA-4, as demonstrated by the phenotype of the CTLA-4 deficient mouse strain, suggests a previously unsuspected means by which costimulation can regulate immune responses, and potentially offers a new means for downregulating activated T-cells by triggering CTLA-4-B7 interactions, or enhancing responses by blocking this inhibitory pathway. Therefore, the B7-CD28/CTLA-4 pathway potentially offers at least two avenues for down-modulating T-cell activation: blockade of T-cell activation through B7-CD28, or triggering B7-CTLA-4 interactions to downregulate activated T-cell mediating autoimmune disease. Conversely, T-cell responses could be enhanced by promoting B7-CD28 interactions (e.g., vaccine approaches for tumors and infectious agents) or by blocking B7-CTLA-4 interactions (e.g., for enhancing anti-tumor immunity). The striking effects of *in vivo* manipulation of this important costimulatory pathway suggest that further understanding of the physiologic functions of the B7-CD28/CTLA-4 costimulatory pathway *in vivo* should facilitate the design of rational therapeutic approaches to manipulate this key immunoregulatory pathway for regulating T-cell activation and self-tolerance.

Acknowledgments
This work was supported by grants form the National Institutes of Health and the Lucille P. Markey Charitable Trust.

References

1. Schwartz, R.H., Mueller, D.L., Jenkins, M.K. and Quill, H. (1989) T-cell clonal anergy. Cold Spring Harb *Symp. Quant. Biol.* 54(1): 605–10.
2. Clark, E.A. and Ledbetter, J.A. (1994) How B and T-cells talk to each other. *Nature* 367: 425–428.
3. Boussiotis, V.A., Gribben, J.G., Freeman, G.J. and Nadler, L.M. (1994) Blockade of the CD28 costimulatory pathway: a means to induce tolerance. *Curr. Opin. Immunol.* 6: 797–807.
4. Lenschow, D.J., Walunas, T.L. and Bluestone, J.A. (1996) CD28/B7 system of T-cell costimulation. *Ann. Rev. Immunol.* 14: 233–58.
5. June, C.H., Bluestone, J.A., Nadler, L.M. and Thompson, C.B. (1994) The B7 and CD28 receptor families. *Immunol. Tod.* 15(7): 321–31.
6. Linsley, P.S. and Golstein, P. (1996) Lymphocyte activation: T-cell regulation by CTLA-4. *Curr. Biol.* 4: 398–400.
7. Tivol, E.A., Borriello, F., Schweitzer, A.N., Lynch, W.P., Bluestone, J.A. and Sharpe, A.H. (1995) Loss of CTLA-4 leads to massive lymphoproliferation and fatal multiorgan tissue destruction, revealing a critical negative regulatory role of CTLA-4. *Immunity* 3: 541–547.
8. Waterhouse, P., Penninger, J.M., Timms, E. et al. (1995) Lymphoproliferative disorders with early lethality in mice deficient in CTLA-4. *Science* 270: 985–988.
9. Constant, S., Schweitzer, N., West, J., Ranney, P. and Bottomly, K. (1995) B lymphocytes can be competent antigen-presenting cells for priming CD4+ T-cells to protein antigens *in vivo*. *J. Immunol.* 155: 3734–3741.
10. Goldstein, M.D. and Watts, T.H. (1996) Identification of distinct domains in CD40 involved in B7-1 induction or growth inhibition. *J. Immunol.* 157: 2837–2843.
11. Miller, S.D., Vanderlugt, C.L., Lenschow, D.J. et al. (1995) Blockade of CD28/B7-1 interaction prevents epitope spreading and clinical relapses of murine EAE. *Immunity* 3: 739–745.

12. Sharpe, A.H. (1996) Costimulatory signals and viral immunity. *Seminars in Virology* 7: 103–111.
13. Freeman, G.J., Boussiotis, V.A., Gribben, J.G., Bernstein, G.M., Gray, G.S. and Nadler, L.M. (1995) B7-1 and B7-2 do not deliver identical costimulatory signals, since B7-2 but not B7-1 preferentially costimulates the initial production of IL-4. *Immunity* 2: 523–532.
14. Kuchroo, V., Prabhu Das, M., Brown, J.A. et al. (1995) B7-1 and B7-2 costimulatory molecules differentially activate the Th1/Th2 developmental pathways: application to autoimmune disease therapy. *Cell* 80: 707–716.
15. Lenschow, D.J., Ho SC, Sattar, H. et al. (1995) Differential effects of anti-B7-1 and anti-B7-2 monoclonal antibody treatment on the development of diabetes in the nonobese diabetic mouse. *J. Exp. Med.* 181: 1145–1155.
16. Gajewski, T.F. (1996) B7-1 but not B7-2 efficiently costimulates CD8$^+$ T lymphocytes in the P815 tumor system *in vitro*. *J. Immunol.* 156(2): 465–472.
17. Lanier, L.L., Ofallon, S., Somoza, C. et al. (1995) CD80 (B7) and CD86(B70) provide similar costimulatory signals for T-cell proliferation, cytokine production, and generation of CTL. *J. Immunol.* 154: 97–105.
18. Schweitzer, A.N., Borriello, F., Wong, R., Abbas, A.K. and Sharpe, A.H. The role of costimulators in T-cell differentiation: Studies using antigen-presenting cells lacking expression of CD80 or CD86. *J. Immunol.* 158: 2713–2722.
19. Mosmann, T.R. and Coffman, R.L. (1989) Th1 and Th2 cells: Different patterns of lymphokine secretion lead to different functional properties. *Ann. Rev. Immunol.* 7: 145–173.
20. Abbas, A.K., Murphy, S.M. and Sher, A. (1996) Functional diversity of helper T lymphocytes. *Nature* 383: 787–793.
21. Seder, R.A. and Paul, W.E. (1994) Acquisition of lymphokine-producing phenotype by CD4$^+$ T-cells. *Ann. Rev. Immunol.* 12: 635–73.
22. Wallace, P.M., Rodgers, J.N., Leytze, G.M., Johnson, J.S. and Linsley, P.S. (1995) Induction and reversal of long-lived specific unresponsiveness to a T-dependent antigen following CTLA4-Ig treatment. *J. Immunol.* 154: 5885–5895.
23. Lu, P., Zhou XD, Chen, S.-J. et al. (1994) CTLA-4 ligands are required to induce an *in vivo* interleukin 4 response to a gastrointestinal nematode parasite. *J. Exp. Med.* 180: 693–8.
24. McKnight, A.J., Perez, V.L., Shea, C.M., Gray, G.S. and Abbas, A.K. (1994) Costimulator dependence of lymphokine secretion by naïve and activated CD4$^+$ T lymphocytes from TCR transgenic mice. *J. Immunol.* 152: 5220–5.
25. Tan, P., Anasetti, C., Hansen, J.A. et al. (1993) Induction of alloantigen-specific hyporesponsiveness in human T lymphocytes by blocking interaction of CD28 with its natural ligand B7/BB1. *J. Exp. Med.* 177: 165–173.
26. Perrin, P.J., Scott, D., Quigley, L. et al. (1995) Role of B7/CD28 CTLA-4 in the induction of chronic relapsing experimental allergic encephalomyelitis. *J. Immunol.* 154: 1481–1490.
27. Corry, D.B., Reiner, S.L., Linsley, P.S. and Locksley, R.M. (1994) Differential effects of blockade of CD28-B7 on the development of Th1 or Th2 effector cells in experimental leishmaniasis. *J. Immunol.* 153: 4142–8.
28. Brown, D.R., Green, J.M., Moskowitz, N.H., Davis, M., Thompson, C.B. and Reiner, S.L. (1996) Limited Role of CD28-mediated signals in T helper subset differentiation. *J. Exp. Med.* 184: 803–810.
29. Boise, L., Minn, A., Noel, P. et al. (1995) CD28 costimulation can promote T-cell survival by enhancing the expression of Bcl-xl. *Immunity* 3: 87–98.
30. Stephens, L. and Kay, T. (1995) Pancreatic expression of B7 costimulatory molecules in the non-obese diabetic mouse. *Int. Immunol.* 7: 1885–1895.
31. Racke, M.K., Scott, D.E., Quigley, L. et al. (1995) Distinct Roles for B7-1 (CD80) and B7-2 (CD86) in the initiation of experimental allergic encephalomyelitis. *J. Clin. Invest.* 96: 2195–2203.
32. Hirokawa, M., Kitabayashi, A., Kuroki, J. and Miura, A.B. (1995) Signal transduction by B7/BB1 expressed on activated T lymphocytes-crosslinking of B7/BB1 induces protein tyrosine phosphorylation and synergizes with signaling through T-cell receptor/CD3. *Immunology* 86: 155–161.
33. Walunas, T.L., Lenschow, D.J., Bakker, C.Y. et al. (1994) CTLA-4 can function as a negative regulator of T-cell activation. *Immunity* 1: 405–413.
34. Gribben, J.G., Freeman, G.J., Boussiotis, V.A. et al. (1994) CTLA4 mediated costimulation induces apoptosis of activated human T lymphocytes. *Proc. Natl. Acad. Sci. USA* 92: 811–815.
35. Krummel, M. and Allison, J.P. (1995) CD28 and CTLA-4 have opposing effects on the response of T-cells to stimulation. *J. Exp. Med.* 182: 459–466.
36. Kearney, E.R., Walunas, T.L., Karr, A.W. et al. (1995) Antigen-dependent clonal expansion of antigen-specific CD4$^+$ T-cells *in vivo* is dependent on CD28 costimulation and inhibited by CTLA-4. *J. Immunol.* 155: 1032–1036.
37. Lane, P., Haller, C. and McConnell, F. (1996) Evidence that induction of tolerance *in vivo* involves active signaling *via* a B7 ligand-dependent mechanism: CTLA4-Ig protects Vb8$^+$ T-cells from tolerance induction by the superantigen staphylococcal enterotoxin B. *Eur. J. Immunol.* 26: 858–862.
38. van Parijs, L. and Abbas, A.K. (1996) Role of Fas-mediated cell death in the regulation of immune responses. *Curr. Opin. Immunol.* 8: 355–361.
39. Leach, D.R., Krummel, M.F. and Allison, J.P. (1996) Enhancement of antitumor immunity by CTLA-4 blockade. *Science* 271: 1734–1736.

40. Karandikar, N., Vanderlugt, C.L., Walunas, T.L., Miller, S.D. and Bluestone, J.A. (1996) CTLA-4: A negative regulator of autoimmune disease. *J. Exp. Med.*; *in press*.
41. Walunas, T.L., Bakker, C.Y. and Bluestone, J.A. (1996) CTLA-4 ligation blocks CD28-dependent T-cell activation. *J. Exp. Med.* 183: 2541–2550.
42. Krummel, M.F. and Allison, J.P. (1996) CTLA-4 engagement inhibits IL-2 accumulation and cell cycle progression upon activation of resting T-cells. *J. Exp. Med.* 183: 2533–2540.
43. Marengere, L.E.M., Waterhouse, P., Duncan, G.D., Mittrucker, H., Feng, G. and Mak, T.W. (1996) Regulation of T-cell receptor signaling by tyrosine phosphatase syp association with CTLA-4. *Science* 272: 1170–1173.
44. Thomas, M.L. (1995) of ITAMS and ITIMS: Turning on and off the B-cell antigen receptor. *J. Exp. Med.* 181: 1953–1955.
45. Turka, L.A., Linsley, P.S., Lin, H. et al. (1992) T-cell activation by the CD28 ligand B7 is required for cardiac allograft rejection *in vivo*. *Proc. Natl. Acad. Sci. USA* 89: 11102–11105.
46. Lenschow, D.J., Zeng, Y., Thistlethwaite, J.R. et al. (1992) Long-term survival of xenogeneic pancreatic islet grafts induced by CTLA4Ig. *Science* 257(5071): 789–792.
47. Harlan, D.M., Abe, R., Lee, K.P. and June, C.H. (1995) Potential Roles of the B7 and CD28 receptor families in autoimmunity and immune evasion. *Clin. Immunol. Immunopathol.* 75: 99–111.
48. Cross, A.H., Girard, T.J., Giacoletto, K.S. et al. (1995) Long-term inhibition of murine experimental autoimmune encephalomyelitis using CTLA4-Fc supports a key role for CD28 costimulation. *J. Clin. Invest.* 95: 2783–2789.

AAS 49
Therapeutic Strategies for Modulating the Inflammatory Diseases
© 1998 Birkhäuser Verlag Basel/Switzerland

Symposium new drugs for inflammatory, allergic and immunologic disease

J.B. Summers[1] and R.D. Dyer[2]

[1]Abbott Laboratories, D4MM AP10, Abbott Park, IL 60064, USA and [2]Parke-Davis Pharmaceutical Research Division, Warner-Lambert Company, 2800 Plymouth Road, Ann Arbor, MI 48105, USA

The Eight International Conference on Inflammation Research concluded with a new symposium format that was designed to feature debut presentations of drugs in the early stages of clinical trials. Presentations that represented late breaking developments in the effort to identify new therapeutic agents were selected only a few weeks prior to the conference. Preference was given to those new drugs which had not been widely reported previously. Speakers were encouraged to provide a comprehensive overview of the preclinical selection and characterization of the drug, evidence for a role of the agent in the treatment of disease and initial clinical results. Presentations that best met the criteria established for the symposium were selected from more than two dozen proposals solicited from the research community.

Dr. Nolan Wood (Roche Products, LTD) opened the symposium with an update on Ro 32-3555, a cartilage protection agent currently involved in clinical trials for the management of arthritis. Ro 32-3555 is an inhibitor of matrix metalloproteinases, which are enzymes widely thought to be a major contributor to joint destruction. Although more than a dozen MMPs have been identified and potentially linked to disease, Roche has chosen to specifically target the collagenases for inhibition. Ro 32-3555 is a selective inhibitor of the collagenase family of MMPs, having IC_{50} values in the low nanomolar range for fibroblast and neutrophil collagenase and collagenase-3, but two orders of magnitude weaker as an inhibitor of stromelysin or gelatinase A. The compound effectively protects cartilage both *in vitro* as demonstrated in an IL-1 induced cartilage explant degradation assay as well as *in vivo* as seen in a cartilage sponge implant model. The drug is well absorbed in rats and marmosets although it is extensively metabolized. Phase I clinical trials with Ro 32-3555 have been completed using doses ranging from 10 to 150 mg in normal human volunteers. The drug was well tolerated with no drug related adverse events or perturbations in clinical chemistries or vital signs. Ro 32-3555 displayed an elimination half life of 21-33 h in man. Food reduced the C_{max} of the drug, but had no significant effect on the area under the curve. Phase II clinical trials in rheumatoid arthritis are underway and Roche also has plans to evaluate the compound in osteoarthritis and tumor metastasis.

Dr. Richard Hubbard (G.D. Searle) described the latest results with celecoxib (SC-58635), a selective cyclooxygenase-2 (Cox-2) inhibitors being developed for the treatment of rheumatoid- and osteo arthritis and other diseases. A substantial amount of preclinical evidence supports the hypothesis that selective inhibition of Cox-2 without significant inhibition of Cox-1 will provide the clinical benefit of traditional non-steroidal antiinflammatory drugs (NSAIDs) without the typical gastrointestinal or kidney side effects. Celecoxib is a 350 fold more potent inhibitor of recombinant human Cox-2 than Cox-1. It is also quite effective in standard inflammation models including rat adjuvant arthritis or carrageenan induced paw edema. Although it inhibits prosta- glandin production in a carrageenan induced air pouch at doses below 1 mg/kg, it produces only a minor inhibition of gastric prostaglandins at 600 mg/kg.

Dr. Hubbard described the results of several clinical trials with celecoxib. When given as a single 100 or 400 mg dose, the drug was as effective as 650 mg aspirin in controlling pain fol- lowing wisdom tooth extraction. In a rheumatoid arthritis trial doses of 200 or 400 mg BID for 4 weeks, provided a significant improvement in morning stiffness, number of painful joints, patient assessed pain score, and withdrawal rate relative to placebo. The magnitude of the effect appeared to be similar to historical results with other NSAIDs. Significant improvement was also seen in an osteoarthritis trial where celecoxib was given at doses of 40, 100, and 200 mg BID for 2 weeks. Trials designed specifically to look at side effect potential were also described. Celecoxib (100 or 200 mg BID for 7 days) produced no ulcers as assessed by endoscopy while Naprosyn (500 mg BID) produced ulcers in 18% of the patients. Gastric erosions were comparable to pla- cebo (about 15%) while approximately 70% of the subjects receiving Naprosyn displayed erosi- ons. Celecoxib also had no effect on platelet function following 400 mg BID for 6 days. Thus the results presented by Dr. Hubbard are consistent with the vision of Cox-2 inhibitors providing a safer yet equally effective alternative to traditional NSAIDs. However, confirmation of these initial findings await more extensive clinical evaluation.

Dr. Satwant Narula (Schering-Plough Research Institute) provided an overview of the precli- nical pharmacology and early clinical results with interleukin-10 (IL-10, SCH-52000). IL-10 is a 18kD cytokine with primarily anti-inflammatory properties. It is produced by T-cells, macropha- ges, B-cells and keratinocytes and causes the reduction in the expression of pro-inflammatory cytokines including TNF-α, IL-1, IL-6 and IL-8 as well as a reduction in ICAM, Cox-2, and iNOS. IL-10 knockout mice display no phenotypic abnormalities in their immune response but develop a severe colitis as they age which has features that resembles both Crohn's and ulcerative colitis. These results have prompted a clinical program using IL-10 for the treatment of inflamma- tory bowel disease.

IL-10 is well tolerated in man and has a half life of 1.1 to 2.5 h. In volunteers that received a low dose LPS challenge, concomitant treatment with IL-10 (1 µg/kg) resulted in a dramatic reduction in IL-1, IL-6, IL-8 and TNF-α blood levels as well as a lower febrile response. Initial trials in steroid refractory Crohn's disease patients demonstrated a 50% response rate to the cytokine. Remission was still present 2 weeks after the end of therapy.

Dr. Louis Renzetti (Hoffman-LaRoche, Inc) described lenercept (Ro 45-2081), an anti tumor necrosis factor approach to the treatment of sepsis. Lenercept is fusion protein linking two extra-membrane components of the human p55 (type I) TNF receptor with the Fc portion of human IgG1. This fusion protein is 50 times more effective inhibitor of TNF than the native soluble receptor alone and 100 fold more effective than a high affinity antibody to TNF. A 20 µg dose of the protein provides complete protection to an LD_{100} LPS challenge. In a baboon bacteremia model lenercept also provided a substantial improvement in survival. Among those animals receiving the drug, 14/16 survived the challenge while only 1 of 8 vehicle treated animals survived. Improvements in mean arterial pressure and reductions in rescue fluid use and pro-inflammatory cytokine levels were also noted. In a phase II clinical trial involving patients with severe sepsis a dose of 0.083 mg/kg was associated with a 36% reduction in 28 day mortality. No effect was seen when treating the more severe refractory shock patients. Further trials in sepsis are ongoing and the use of lenercept in other inflammatory diseases is being considered.

Dr. David Snyder (Eli Lilly) provided an update on LY-315, 920 a potent inhibitor of synovial phospholipase A_2 (sPLA_2). The primary focus of the LY-315, 920 development program is in the treatment of sepsis where sPLA_2 blood levels are elevated by 200–500 fold. Dr. Snyder also reported results from the use of a baboon bacteremia model. A 3 mg/kg bolus dose of LY-315, 920 followed by a constant infusion of 0.5 mg/kg/h resulted in a complete inhibition of sPLA_2 activity in the blood and a 50% improvement in survival relative to the untreated control animals. The extent of ARDS and disseminated intravascular coagulation seen in the treated baboons was less than seen in the controls. Initial phase I trials have been completed with LY-315, 920 using a single 30-minute infusion of the drug. A half-life of about 5 h was observed.

AAS 49
Therapeutic Strategies for Modulating the Inflammatory Diseases
© 1998 Birkhäuser Verlag Basel/Switzerland

Cartilage protective agent (CPA) Ro 32-3555, a new matrix metalloproteinase inhibitor for the treatment of rheumatoid arthritis

N.D. Wood, M. Aitken, S. Durston, S. Harris, G.R. McClelland and S. Sharp

Roche Products Ltd, Broadwater Road, Welwyn Garden City, Hertfordshire, AL7 3AY, UK

Summary. CPA was well tolerated at all dose levels (10–150 mg) following single oral dose administration to healthy male volunteers. There was no relationship between the intensity, duration and number of adverse events reported and the dose of CPA. There was a dose-related increase in exposure as measured by $AUC_{0-\infty}$ and C_{max}. Administration of 10 mg CPA following food resulted in a delayed t_{max}, and a significant decrease in C_{max} but not $AUC_{0-\infty}$.

Introduction

Rheumatoid arthritis (RA) is a chronic systemic inflammatory disease affecting approximately 1 % of the adult population. The prominent features of the disease include synovial cell proliferation and destruction of the adjacent articular cartilage in the affected joint [1]. Current therapies are directed towards the various components of the chronic inflammatory response and often involve the simultaneous administration of several drugs. However, these therapies are not always specific and they often fail. Non-steroidal anti-inflammatory drugs (NSAIDs) provide symptomatic relief, but do not decrease the rate of cartilage degradation or alter the course of the disease. Similarly, although the disease modifying anti-rheumatic drugs (DMARDs) offer initial control, they are often difficult to use long-term because of side-effects and flares in disease activity [2]. Recent advances in the understanding of the aetiology and pathogenesis of RA have led to the development of new therapies based on inhibition of a specific pathophysiological component of the disease. Development of the cartilage protective agent (CPA) is an example of this approach [3, 4].

Articular cartilage is a highly specialised tissue, the integrity of which is critical for the protection of the underlying bone and smooth articulation of the joint. It is a fibre-reinforced composite matrix, the principal structural components of which are proteoglycan and type II collagen. The hydrophilic characteristics of the proteoglycan molecules induce a swelling pressure within the cartilage which allows it to resist compressive forces, while the type II collagen network provides its tensile strength and load distribution properties [5]. In pathological conditions such as RA, there is an initial net loss of the proteoglycan matrix. However, this step is reversible providing the supporting collagen network remains intact. It is the subsequent destruction of the collagen network which is regarded as the key irreversible step resulting in the integrity of the matrix being destroyed and the loss of articular cartilage [6].

Cartilage degradation results from the synergistic action of the matrix metalloproteinases (MMPs) collagenases, stromelysins, gelatinases and others. Under normal physiological conditions, control of these enzymes is exerted at several levels [7]. Ordinarily, matrix synthesis is finely balanced by controlled matrix degradation. In RA, increased MMP activity in response to inflammatory stimuli such as Interleukin-1 and tumour necrosis factor leads to accelerated cartilage destruction [8]. Collagenases are the only enzymes capable of cleaving triple helical collagen at physiological pHs. This cleavage occurs at a single well-characterised amide bond and provides a good target for therapeutic intervention. CPA, a novel orally bioavailable collagenase inhibitor developed from a knowledge of the collagen cleavage site, has been shown to prevent cartilage destruction both *in vitro* and *in vivo* [9, 10]. CPA may therefore prevent the progressive structural joint damage which is thought to be associated with loss of joint function and pain in RA patients. This paper reports the tolerability and pharmacokinetics following the administration of single ascending oral doses of CPA to healthy male volunteers. This was the first human administration of this compound.

Methods

Forty-eight healthy male volunteers, aged 21–49 years, participated in the study. All subjects gave written informed consent before screening assessments and the protocol was approved by the local Independent Ethics Committee. The study was a double-blind, placebo-controlled single ascending oral dose study in which subjects were allocated to groups of 8 per dose level and randomised to receive either CPA (n=6) or placebo (n=2). CPA was administered at doses of 10, 25, 50, 75, 100 and 150 mg as an aqueous oral drinking solution following an overnight fast. Subjects randomised to placebo received an equivalent volume of solution of identical appearance and taste. The decision to escalate the dose was based on a blinded review of safety, tolerability and pharmacokinetic data for at least four subjects at the preceding dose. After dose escalation had been completed, subjects who had received 10 mg CPA or placebo returned to receive a second dose following a standardised breakfast. Subjects remained in the investigational unit for 24 h after all doses. Consumption of alcohol or smoking was not allowed on the study day and subjects were confined to their beds until 4 h post-dose. A light lunch was provided 4 h after dosing and an evening meal 10 h after dosing.

Blood samples for pharmacokinetic analysis were collected before dosing and at intervals up to 96 h post-dose. Due to the rapid absorption observed following the first (10 mg) dose, additional blood samples were taken at 10 and 20 minutes post-dose for all subsequent groups. Blood pressure and heart rate were measured with the subjects in a semi-supine position using automated devices and continuous lead II ECG monitoring was performed for the first 4 h post-dose (Spacelab Heart Monitors). Twelve-lead ECG recordings were taken pre-dose and at regular intervals up to 24 h post-dose (Hewlett Packard PageWriter). Adverse events were monitored continuously throughout the study. In addition, blood samples were taken for clinical laboratory tests before and after each dose.

Plasma concentrations of CPA were measured using a specific HPLC-MS-MS method after extraction on C8 Bond-elut cartridges. Extracted samples were then transferred to autosampler vials and injected onto a Phenomenex Ultracarb5 ODS column (30×4.6 mm i.d.) and eluted using a mobile phase of 80% acetonitrile in 2.5 mM ammonium formate (pH3) at a flow rate of 1.0 ml/min. Selective detection was accomplished on a Sciex (API 111 plus) mass spectrometer in the multiple reaction monitoring mode using atmospheric pressure chemical ionisation. The calibration range was 0.5–200 ng/ml and the mean inter-assay precision on standards and quality control samples was $\pm 8.1\%$ and $\pm 12.6\%$ respectively.

Pharmacokinetic parameters were derived by non-compartmental methods using Topfit (version 2.0). The observed peak plasma concentration (C_{max}) and the time taken to reach peak concentration (t_{max}) were taken directly from the plasma-concentration time profiles. The area under the plasma concentration-time curve was estimated by the linear trapezoidal rule up to the last measurable concentration (Ct) and extrapolated to infinity ($AUC_{0-\infty}$) by the addition of Ct/λz where λz is the terminal elimination rate constant obtained by log-linear regression. The elimination half-life ($t_·$) was calculated by $\ln(2)/\lambda z$. Mean dose-normalised values of C_{max} and $AUC_{0-\infty}$ were compared by analysis of variance (ANOVA) to test for dose-proportionality. Paired t-Tests on the geometric means of C_{max} and $AUC_{0-\infty}$ were performed to test for the effect of food on the pharmacokinetics of CPA.

Results and discussion

CPA was well tolerated at all dose levels. There were no serious adverse events. The most common adverse events were local bruising, headache and nasopharyngitis. All reports of bruising were described as either secondary to insertion of the cannula for blood sampling or following venepuncture. A summary of adverse events according to treatment group is given in Table 1.

Most adverse events were of mild intensity. One subject experienced severe back pain approximately 24 days after receiving a dose of 10 mg CPA under fasted conditions. The event occurred as the subject lifted a patient whilst going about his daily duties as an ambulance driver.

Table 1. Summary of adverse events

	Placebo (n=12)	10 mg[a] (n=6)	25 mg (n=6)	50 mg (n=6)	75 mg (n=6)	100 mg n=6)	150 mg (n=6)
Number of subjects with 1 or more AE	9	6	4	3	3	2	3
Number of AES	13	11	5	3	4	5	4

[a] Five of six subjects received 10 mg CPA on two separate occasions (before and after food)

It was therefore considered unrelated to treatment. The subject returned as planned to complete the effect of food arm of the study. There was no apparent relationship between the intensity, duration and number of adverse events reported and the dose of CPA.

Approximately 4 h after receiving 10 mg CPA under fasted conditions, one subject experienced transient ventricular tachycardia (a run of seven beats in sequence) lasting approximately 2 seconds. The event was detected during routine lead II ECG monitoring. The subject was asymptomatic and went on to complete all assessments, however he was excluded from the effect of food arm of the study. The ECG rhythm strip was reviewed by an external consultant cardiologist who concluded that the event was probably benign. The event was not considered related to study drug as it occurred 4 h after the lowest dose of CPA and was not observed at any other dose level. There were no clinically relevant changes in vital signs, clinical laboratory parameters or 12-lead ECG recordings at any dose.

Under fasted conditions, CPA was rapidly absorbed. This was followed by an initial rapid decline phase and a slow terminal elimination phase. Mean plasma concentration-time profiles for the 10, 50 and 150 mg dose groups are illustrated in Figure 1.

The mean half-life associated with the terminal elimination phase ranged from 21–33 h, suggesting that once daily dosing may be adequate for future studies. There was a 2–4 fold variability in C_{max} and $AUC_{0-\infty}$ between subjects, although individual subject plasma concentration-time profiles were similar in shape at all dose levels (Fig. 1).

As predicted from the animal data [10], both C_{max} and $AUC_{0-\infty}$ increased with dose. ANOVA after logarithmic transformation of the dose-normalised mean data revealed no relevant deviation from dose-proportionality (C_{max} $p=0.820$; $AUC_{0-\infty}$ $p=0.156$).

The mean ± s.d. pharmacokinetic parameters of CPA following single oral dose administration to healthy male volunteers are summarised in Table 2.

Administration of 10 mg CPA following a standardised breakfast resulted in a delay in tmax, a significant reduction in C_{max}, but no effect on $AUC_{0-\infty}$. Values of C_{max} before and after food were 286±94 ng/ml and 130±31 ng/ml respectively ($p=0.011$; paired t-test), with corres-

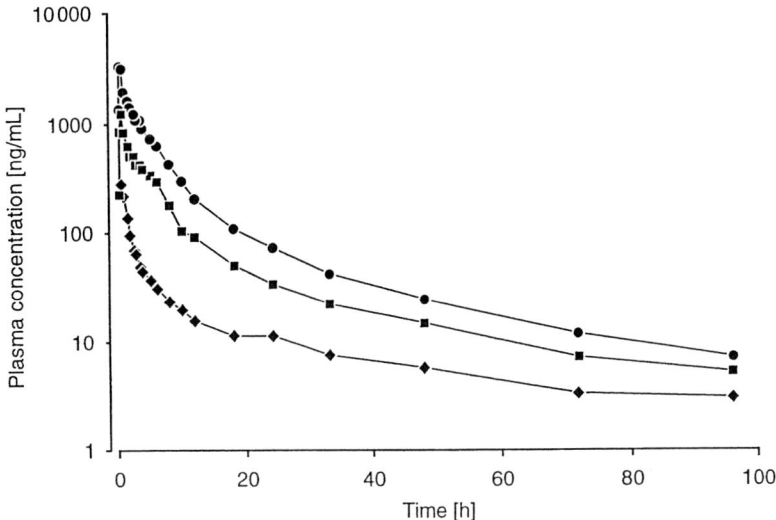

Figure 1. Mean plasma concentration-time profiles of 10 (◆), 50 (■) and 150 mg (●) CPA following single oral dose administration to healthy male volunteers (n=6).

Table 2. Mean ± s.d. pharmacokinetic parameters of CPA following single oral dose administration to healthy male volunteers

Dose[a] (mg)	C_{max} (ng/ml)	t_{max} (h)	$AUC_{0-\infty}$ (mg.h/l)	t· (h)
10	286±94	0.67±0.26	1.30±0.47	29.7±6.3
10 + Food	130±31	1.40±0.82	1.13±0.29	32.6±3.3
25	805±460	0.83±0.41	4.28±2.40	24.5±4.9
50	1272±321	0.56±0.23	6.14±2.12	24.4±3.0
75	1714±272	0.56±0.23	7.35±1.42	21.2±3.3
100	2456±973	0.53±0.25	10.67±6.49	24.0±2.4
150	3484±1228	0.39±0.09	13.31±4.86	25.0±2.5

[a] n=6 for all groups except 10 + Food where n=5

ponding t_{max} values of 0.67±0.2 h and 1.40±0.82 h. $AUC_{0-\infty}$ values before and after food were 1.30±0.47 mg.h/l and 1.13±0.29 mg.h/l respectively (p=0.577; paired t-test). The mean plasma concentration time-profiles following the administration of 10 mg CPA before and after food are shown in Figure 2.

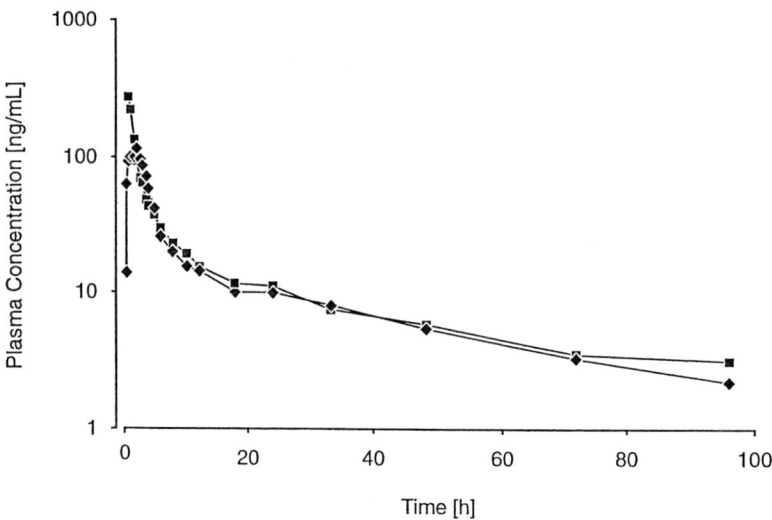

Figure 2. Mean plasma concentration-time profiles of CPA following single oral doses of 10 mg to healthy male volunteers before food (■ n=6) and after food (◆ n=5).

In conclusion, CPA was well tolerated at all dose levels in this healthy volunteer study with no relationship between the number of adverse events reported and the dose of CPA. There was a dose-related increase in exposure as assessed by C_{max} and $AUC_{0-\infty}$. Administration of CPA following food resulted in a significant reduction in C_{max} but not $AUC_{0-\infty}$. The long terminal elimination phase half-life suggests once daily dosing may be adequate.

References

1. Harris, E.D. (1990) Rheumatoid arthritis; Pathophysiology and implications for therapy. *N. Engl. J. Med.* 322: 1277–1289.
2. Brooks, P.M. (1993) Clinical management of rheumatoid arthritis. *Lancet* 341: 286–290.
3. Westmacott, D., Bradshaw, D., Kumar, M.K.H., Lewis, E.J., Murray, E.J., Nixon, J.S. and Sedgwick, A.D. (1991) Molecular basis of new approaches to the therapy of rheumatoid arthritis. *Molecular aspects of medicine* 12: 395–473.
4. Vincenti, M.P., Clark, I.M. and Brinckerhoff, C.E. (1994) Using inhibitors of metalloproteinases to treat arthritis. *Arthritis Rheum.* 37: 1115–1126.
5. Hardingham, T.E., Venn, G. and Bayliss, M.T. (1991) Chondrocyte responses in cartilage and experimental osteoarthritis. *Brit. J. Rheumatol.* 30 (Suppl. 1): 32–37.
6. Jubb, R.W. and Fell, H.B. (1980) The breakdown of collagen by chondrocytes. *J. Pathol.* 130: 159–167.
7. Murphy, G. (1995) Matrix metalloproteinases and their inhibitors. *Acta Orthop. Scand.* 66 (Suppl. 266): 55–60.
8. Krane, S.M., Amento, E.P., Goldring, M.B., Goldring, S.R. and Stephenson, M.L. (1988) Modulation of matrix synthesis and degradation in join inflammation. *In:* A.M. Galvert (ed.): *Research Monographs in Cell and Tissue Physiology.* Elsevier, Amsterdam, pp 179–195.

9. Johnson, W.H., Roberts, N.A., Borkakoti, N. (1987) Collagenase inhibitors; their design and potential thera-peutic use. *J. Enzyme Inhib.* 2: 1–22.
10. Lewis, E.J., Bishop, J., Bottomley, K.M.K., Bradshaw, D., Brown, P.A., Broadhurst, M.J., Budd, J.M., Elliott, L., Gibson, V.M., Greenham, A.K., Hill, C.H., Johnson, W.H., Lawton, G., Nixon, J.S., Rose, F. and Sutton, B. Ro 32-3555 (Cartilage Protective Agent), an orally active collagenase inhibitor prevents cartilage breakdown *in vitro* and *in vivo. Brit. J. Pharmacol.* 121: 540–546.

AAS 49
Therapeutic Strategies for Modulating the Inflammatory Diseases
© 1998 Birkhäuser Verlag Basel/Switzerland

Immunomodulation of Crohn's disease by Interleukin-10

S.K. Narula, D. Cutler and P. Grint

Schering-Plough Research Institute, 2015 Galloping Hill Road, Kenilworth, NJ 07033, USA

Summary. Interleukin-10 is an important cytokine that is involved in regulation of pro-inflammatory cytokines and T-cell responses. Interleukin-10 has been studied extensively in various preclinical and clinical models of inflammation. The most remarkable and consistently reproducible quality of IL-10 is its ability to downregulate macrophage functions. This includes inhibiting the production of pro-inflammatory cytokines such TNF-α, Interleukin-1, Interleukin-6 and antigen presentation by these professional antigen presenting cells. Additionally, Interleukin-10 also has effects on various other cell types of hematopoietic origin such as B-cells, neutrophils, and most importantly T-cells. Interleukin-10 has shown efficacy in several models of autoimmune disease. The present article deals with the effect of Interleukin-10 in animal models of inflammatory bowel disease and the results of phase I clinical trials in normal human volunteers and chronic active Crohn's disease patients.

Introduction

Helper T-cell populations have been studied extensively in both murine and human systems. The two major T helper subsets, viz., Th1 and Th2 are typically defined by the cytokine secretion profile. Th1 cells produce Interleukin 2, Interferon γ and Lymphotoxin. Th2 cells on the other hand secrete IL-4, IL-5 and IL-10. Although it is rapidly becoming evident that the T-cell helper subsets are far more complex than this simple picture, the discovery of IL-10 was a result of studies aimed at studying the cross-regulation of these two major T-cell helper subsets. IL-1, originally termed Cytokine Synthesis Inhibition Factor (CSIF) was discovered as a product of Mouse Th2 clones on the basis of its ability to inhibit IFN-γ synthesis by mouse Th1 clones [1]. The mouse CSIF was cloned in 1988, followed soon thereafter with the cloning of the human homolog [2, 3]. Interestingly, IL-10 has striking homology to the open reading frame BCRF1 of Epstein Barr virus. Although not formally proven, this is considered to be another incident of "cellular gene hijacking" by a virus to evade immune surveillance. The availability of the recombinant material expedited the rapid biological characterization of this cytokine over the next several years. CSIF was renamed Interleukin-10. The receptor was identified and cloned. It was shown to be a member of Interferon family of receptors.

Biological characterization of IL-10

The biological activities of IL-10 have already been described in several reviews that have been published to date on this subject [4–13]. The original studies with IL-10 had already indicated the CSIF activity of Interleukin was totally dependent on the presence of antigen presenting cells. As such, some of the first studies carried out with IL-10 were targeted towards unraveling its activity on macrophages, the "professional" APCs. It was discovered that IL-10 can dramatically downregulate the "monokine cascade" induced in activated monocytes. It strongly downregulated production of pro-inflammatory cytokines such as TNF-α, IL-1 and IL-6. Additionally, the expression of MHC Class II antigens, HLA-DR, -DP and -DQ were markedly downregulated by IL-10. In addition to above, the expression of CD80 and CD86, the ligands for the T-cell co-stimulatory activation pathway are also downregulated. Other important adhesion molecules such as ICAM-I, which are involved in macrophage-T-cell cognate interactions are also downregulated. The fact that IL-10 is a strong regulator of inflammation is evident from the fact that the synthesis of distal inflammatory mediators such as nitric oxide and prostaglandins is also downregulated at the enzyme synthesis level. In fact, the effect of IL-10 is dramatic enough to result in actual morphological reversion of activated macrophages to inactivated appearance. This "deactivation" of

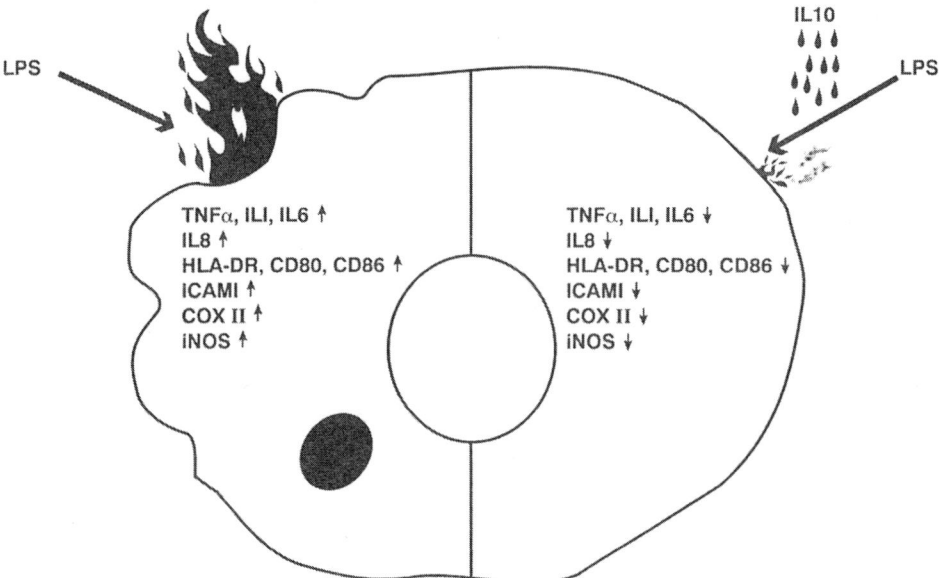

Figure 1. Macrophage deactivation by Interleukin-10.

macrophages leads to an inhibition of antigen presentation and the subsequent activation of T-cells. This can be readily demonstrated in *in vitro* assays by lack of IL-2 production and inhibition of T-cell proliferation (Fig. 1).

Although IL-10 was originally discovered as a product of Th2 helper T-cell clones, it soon became evident that the production of IL-10 was not strictly restricted to this subtype. IL-10 was found to be produced by Human Th0, Th1, Th2 clones as well as activated peripheral blood lymphocytes. IL-10 can also be produced by activated B-cells, UV induced keratinocytes, microglial cells and activated macrophages, where it has been shown to be autoregulatory. In fact, the effects of IL-10 on T-cells are also not entirely mediated through APCs alone. It has been demonstrated that IL-10 can have direct effects on T-cells leading to an inhibition of IL-2 production by Human T-cells. Similarly, the inhibitory effects of IL-10 may not be limited to Th1 cytokines either, since IL-4 and IL-5 can also be inhibited. The effect of IL-10 on CD8$^+$ T-cells may in fact be quite the opposite. IL-10 has been shown to be a proliferation and differentiation factor for murine Cytotoxic lymphocytes and has been shown to promote CD8$^+$ chemotaxis in the human system. In addition to T-cells and macrophages, IL-10 also affects several other cell types. It has been shown to be capable of proliferating activated B-cells. The MHC Class II expression on B-cells is not downregulated by IL-10. IL-10 has also been shown to have an inhibitory effect on the capacity

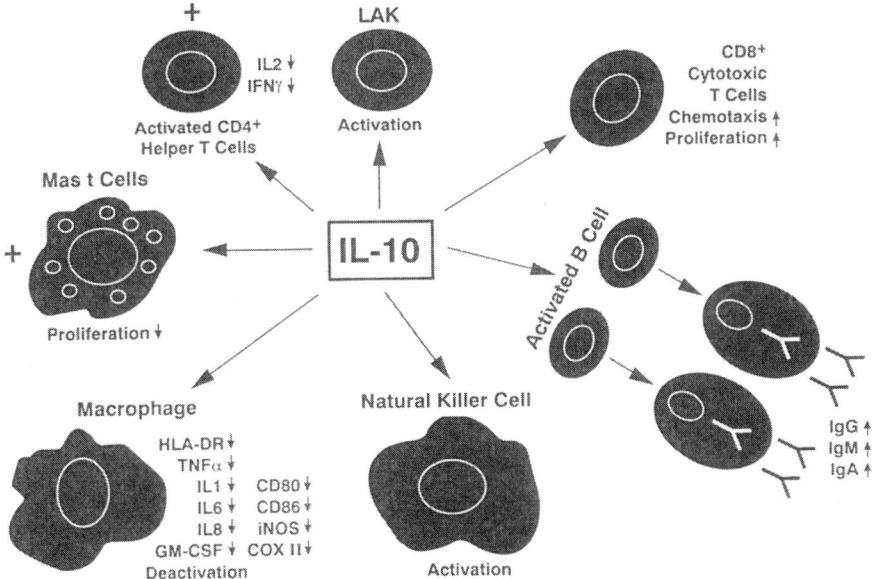

Figure 2. Biological activities of IL-10.

of neutrophils to produce IL-8, a CXC type chemokine. Neutrophils also lose their ability to phagocytose and kill opsonized yeast. IL-10 can also activate NK cells in the presence of IL-2.

Thus, based on several of its *in vitro* activities, IL-10 can be considered a pleiotropic cytokine (Fig. 2). However, the most convincing and consistent *in vivo* activity of IL-10 so far has been its anti-inflammatory activity. This was confirmed by several different laboratories in various murine models of inflammation such as the endotoxin and SEB mediated lethal shock. In these studies IL-10 successfully prevented the production of TNF-α, IL-1 and IL-6. Additionally, it had a marked effect on the survival of the animals. To date, IL-10 has shown efficacy in various models of Arthritis, Experimental Autoimmune Encephalitis, Experimental Autoimmune Thyroiditis, HSV Keratitis, Endotoxin induced uveitis and inflammatory bowel disease models. Since the major focus of this article is on Crohn's disease, data from these studies alone will be discussed here.

Effect of IL-10 in murine models of inflammatory bowel disease

Most of the animal models for inflammatory bowel disease such as the ones induced by acetic acid, TNBS, dextran sulfate, exhibit acute mucosal inflammation but do not represent the human disease which has a chronic relapsing nature. As such, they are not suitable for studying a drug whose mechanism of action may lie in the modulation of immune cells perpetrating a chronic state. IL-10 has been studied in many of these models with varying degrees of success, but mostly it has shown disappointing activities. However, in models which are based on immunological manifestations of the disease, IL-10 has shown remarkable and unmistakable activity.

IL-10 knockout mouse

One of the most effective methodologies available today to define seminal activities of genes is the gene knockout technology. Mice with inactivated IL-10 gene were produced to evaluate the impact of this cytokine on the immune system. Preliminary examination did not yield any specific phenotype. The mice were normal in their T and B-cell responses. Hematopoeisis was normal in these mice and there was no difference in the numbers or distribution of circulating mature cells. However, as the mice aged, they became anemic, lost weight and died prematurely. The major reason for this was development of chronic enterocolitis. Donna Rennick with colleagues at DNAX and SPRI has studied this phenomenon extensively [14–16]. The fact that this condition manifested in specific pathogen free environment lent credence to the hypothesis that endogenous IL-10 plays a regulatory role in suppressing the ongoing intestinal inflammatory response to enteric antigens. In fact, high levels of TNF-α and IFN-γ were detected in intestinal explants of these mice with IL-4 being undetectable. This cytokine profile, although less severe, was also detected in peripheral tissues. When housed under conventional conditions, the disease manifestation was accompanied by histological alterations reminiscent of the human disease. The spleens of these animals had very low levels of red blood cells but were packed with myeloid cells. The mesenteric lymph nodes were similarly enlarged. The intestinal pathology resembled some of the features seen in Crohn's disease. The lesions were scattered throughout the large and small intestine. The mucosal architecture was abnormal and the intestinal walls were thickened. Inflammatory infiltrates were found both around sites of hypoplasia and hyperplasia. These infiltrates had abnormally high levels of CD4$^+$, αβTCR$^+$ and CD4$^+$, CD8$^+$, αβTCR$^+$ activated memory T-cells. Treatment of these animals with antibodies to either TNF-α, IFN-γ or IL-6 diminished the disease, but did not totally ablate it. In fact, none of these antibody treatments could prevent the onset of disease in young animals. IL-10, in contrast to the antibodies showed a significant effect. The animals gained weight and were normal in their development. Histological examination showed reduction in intestinal inflammation. Furthermore, IL-10 could completely prevent the disease in young weanlings. This data demonstrates that the pathogenesis of disease in these animals is due to the activity of several different inflammatory cytokines. Since IL-10 can inhibit most of them simultaneously, it shows superior activity in this model in contrast to the individual antibodies directed against the various cytokines.

The IL-10 -/- mouse has been studied extensively for its responses towards various antigens, especially in extra-intestinal tissues. Results from these studies indicate that although IL-10 may not be absolutely essential for the generation of Th2 cells, it is required for the inhibition of Th1 cells. Both the Delayed Type Hypersensitivity response and contact hypersensitivity is highly exaggerated in these animals. Based on these findings, it is fair to say that an important endogenous role for IL-10 is to control the local production of inflammatory cytokines.

The CD45RB^{hi} model of inflammatory bowel disease

The phenomenon of cross-regulation between CD45RB^{hi} and CD45RB^{lo} CD4 Helper T-cells was discovered within the context of studying Leishmaniasis models. CD45RB^{hi} cells produce IFN-γ whereas CD45RB^{lo} cells produce IL-4. Transfer of CD45RB^{hi} into SCID mice produces a severe colitis in these animals. The disease develops 3 to 4 weeks after T-cell transfer. The inflammation involved the large intestine with involvement of cecum, colon and rectum. Both the mucosal and submucosal layers were infiltrated by predominantly CD4$^+$ cells and macrophages. Extensive epithelial hyperplasia accompanied by loss of mucin producing cells and ulcers with deep fissures were also frequently seen. T-cells from the colons of CD45RB^{hi}-SCID mice have high levels of IFN-γ but have very low to undetectable levels of IL-4 and IL-10. Co-injection of CD45RB^{lo} T-cells could prevent the induction of disease [17].

Treatment with both anti-TNF-α and anti-IFN-γ antibody could prevent the induction of the disease. Combination of the two antibodies, however, did not provide a significant benefit over the individual antibody treatment. Neither of these treatments, however, were as effective as the protection achieved by transfer of CD45RB^{lo} T-cells. Animals treated with IL-10 were totally protected, as the incidence of colitis was identical to that of the control group. Moreover, treatment with IL-10 showed a reduction in the mRNA levels of both IFN-γ and TNF-α. Additionally, histologically, the IL-10 treated mice were totally clear of any inflammation. The disease, however, reappeared on cessation of treatment in all of these cases. Interestingly, IL-4 has no effect on the course of the disease [18].

PG-PS induced granulomatous enterocolitis: Cell walls (peptidoglycan-polysaccharide polymers) of enteric bacteria can induce acute inflammation in susceptible hosts such as Lewis rats that proceeds into a relapsing, granulomatous inflammatory reaction in several organs. The disease is induced by subserosal injection of the PG-PS complex into the terminal ileum and cecum. Acute Inflammation apparent in 1–3 days is characterized by focal intestinal wall thickening, adhesions and mild arthritis. The acute inflammation which is typified by a neutrophil and macrophage infiltrate resolves in 10–14 days but is followed by a T-cell dependent reactivation accompanied by extensive granulomatous bowel inflammation, liver granulomas and arthritis. Both IL-1RA and cyclosporine can attenuate various aspects of the disease, indicating an important role of both IL-1 and T-cells in the development of the disease.

The effect of IL-10 on both the acute and chronic phase of this disease was tested. IL-10 was effective in downregulating inflammation in both the acute and chronic phase of the disease, however, its effects were more pronounced in the chronic phase of the disease. Continuous IL-10 treatment significantly improved gross, histologic, and immunologic parameters of intestinal inflammation. In the chronic phase, the histologic improvement was accompanied by a downregulation of tissue gene expression of IFN-γ, IL-1 and TNF-α. IL-10 also demonstrated dramatic effects on the extra-intestinal manifestations in this model. This was true both in the development of hepatic granulomas and arthritis, both of which were minimally apparent after IL-10 treatment [19].

Since the effect of steroids has been studied in the PG-PS model, it was interesting to carry out combination studies with steroids in this model to evaluate the efficacy of this combination. Preliminary data clearly indicates that there are no adverse effects of using this combination in this model. Indeed, the combination gives a far superior efficacy over either agent alone (manuscript in preparation). This bodes well for the possible use of IL-10 as a steroid sparing agent in the clinical treatment of IBD.

Clinical status of IL-10

Based on the animal safety data, it was determined that IL-10 could be initially tested for safety and tolerance in a normal human volunteer population. The initial studies were designed to investigate the safety, tolerance, pharmacokinetics, subset modulation and cytokine modulation by IL-10. These studies were initially carried out in normal human volunteers. Single dose bolus intravenous injections were administered to groups of patients in a sequentially rising doses. The doses ranged from 0.1 to 100 µg/kg. There were no serious adverse effects. Mild headache, nausea and low-grade fever at 50 and 100 µg/kg doses. Administration of IL-10 was followed by a dose-related monocytosis evident at 6–24 h and a transient reduction in lymphocytes. The LPS induced inflammatory cytokine production in the whole blood from IL-10 treated subjects was dramatically down-regulated, compared to the placebo group. Soluble TNFRI and II were significantly increased. *Ex vivo* proliferative response of T-cells to PHA was also significantly reduced. These effects of IL-10 were evident in doses as low as 1 µg/kg. In the higher dose groups (25 µg/kg and up), effect of IL-10 persisted for up to 48 h in varying degrees depending on the dose group, despite the absence of measurable IL-10 in the serum. This despite the fact that the serum half-life determined from these studies was calculated to be around 1.5–3 h. Importantly, administration of IL-10 also results in a down-regulation of MHC Class II antigen HLA-DR *in vivo*.

The data generated from these studies formed the basis for testing of IL-10 in a sublethal endotoxemia model in normal human volunteers. Administration of 4 ng/kg dose of LPS in humans induces a very well defined "cytokine cascade" which is characterized by sequential appearance of TNF-α, IL-1 and IL-6 and IL-8 with TNF-α levels reaching a peak at 90 min. Doses of IL-10 ranging from 1 µg/kg to 25 µg/kg were tested, where IL-10 was given IV bolus 2 min prior to LPS injection. The outcome of this study bore out the *in vitro* and *in vivo* preclinical findings. IL-10 very clearly demonstrated its ability to inhibit LPS induced TNF-α, IL-1 and IL-6, IL-8 and IL-12 levels *in vivo*. Plasma cortisol level was lower as was peak and average body temperature. All doses tested appeared equally effective. IL-10 also resulted in decreased pulmonary sequestration of neutrophils in response to LPS. Administration of IL-10 (25 µg/kg) 1 h after LPS challenge to healthy volunteers still demonstrated immunomodulatory activity though this activity was not as dramatic as that seen when IL-10 was administered at the same time as the LPS challenge.

The clinical safety of single dose IL-10 administration allowed the testing and confirmation of several of IL-10's activities derived from *in vitro* and animal model studies. One of the seminal activities of IL-10 that provides the rationale for its use in chronic inflammatory disease is its ability to downregulate DTH. This was tested clinically by subjecting patients to a multi-antigen test. In each subject, IL-10 was injected in one arm near the site of antigen test, while the contra-lateral arm was injected with the placebo near the antigen challenge site. IL-10 had a dose-depen-dent effect on inhibiting the DT response. Interestingly, at high doses, the control arm also showed decreased DTH response activity indicating systemic activity of IL-10.

The data derived from these initial clinical studies and the existing animal model data provided further impetus for testing IL-10 in Inflammatory bowel disease. A phase I study was therefore designed to test IL-10 in Chronic Active Crohn's Disease. The primary objective of the study was to test safety and tolerance of IL-10 when given as an IV bolus injection for 7 consecutive days. The trial was designed as a randomized, placebo-controlled, double blind, multiple center trial. The secondary objective was to obtain pharmacodynamic information such as cytokine levels in blood, in pre- and post-treatment biopsy samples, CDAI scores and endoscopic exami-nation. The dosing was once again sequential and ranged from 0.5 µg/kg to 25 µg/kg. IL-10 was safe and well-tolerated, with all patients in the active drug group completing the entire course. The most interesting effect was seen on the CDAI scores of these patients. In 50% of the patients in the IL-10 treated group, improvement in CDAI scores that define remission were observed. Interestingly, this remission was still apparent 2 weeks after cessation of IL-10 treatment. Addi-tionally, the cytokine levels from the biopsy samples also showed a trend towards a decrease in TNF-α and IL-1 levels. Given the initial very positive data from these clinical studies, clinical testing of IL-10 in various chronic inflammatory diseases has been initiated. Ongoing studies include a 28 day subcutaneous dosing in steroid refractory CD patients, 28 day subcutaneous dosing in Chronic active Crohn's Disease patients, 28 day subcutaneous dosing in Ulcerative Colitis, 28 day Subcutaneous dosing in Rheumatoid Arthritis and a 7 day multiple dosing study in normal human volunteers.

Conclusion

The underlying immunopathogenesis of Inflammatory Bowel Disease is already being unraveled. The experience with anti-inflammatory drugs has been disappointing, in that they cannot induce or maintain remissions effectively. Hard-hitting immunosuppressives have toxic liabilities for long-term use and as such, are of limited utility. Disease-specific drugs that can reset the immune system are the ideal therapeutics. In reality, the fine-tuned homeostasis of the human immune response may not lend itself readily to manipulation from without. Endogenous regulators of inflammatory responses such as IL-10 and TGF-β are produced in response to specific stimuli in a local environment. Their eventual effects are dictated by the milieu of cytokines, chemokines and other mediators, including the tissue type. As such, the challenge of converting these endogenous regulators into human therapeutics is not trivial. Our clinical program has at every stage included extensive immunological characterization, in an attempt to use this endogenous regulator in a pragmatic and smart manner. Besides IBD, Interleukin is currently in clinical trials for rheumatoid arthritis and multiple sclerosis.

References

1. Fiorentino, D.F., Bond, M.W. and Mosmann, T.R. (1989) Two types of mouse helper T-cell. IV. Th2 clones secrete a factor that inhibits cytokine production by Th1 clones. *J. Exp. Med.* 170: 2081–2095.
2. Mosmann, T.R., Cherwinski, H., Bond, M.W., Giedlin, M.A. and Coffman, R.L. (1986) Two types of murine helper T-cell clones: 1. Definition according to profiles of lymphokine activities and secreted proteins. *J. Immunol.* 136: 2357–2384.
3. Moore, K.W., Vieira, P., Fiorentino, D.R., Trounstine, M.L., Khan, T.A. and Mosmann, T.R. (1990) Homology of the cytokine synthesis inhibitory factor (IL-10) to the Epstein Barr virus gene BCRF1. *Science* 248: 1230–1234.
4. deWaal Malefyt, R., Yssel, H., Roncarolo, M.-G., Spits, H. and deVries, J.E. (1992) Interleukin 10. *Curr. Opin. Immunol.* 4: 314–320.
5. Spits, H. and deWaal Malefyt, R. (1992) Functional characterization of human IL-10. *Int. Arch. Allergy Immunol.* 99: 8–15.
6. Moore, K.W., O'Garra, A., deWaal Malefyt, R., Vieira, P. and Mosmann, T.R. (1993) Interleukin-10. *Ann. Rev. Immunol.* 11: 165–190.
7. Mosmann, T.R. (1994) Interleukin 10. *In: The Cytokine Handbook,* 2nd Edition, Academic Press Ltd, pp 223–237.
8. Mosmann, T.R. (1994) Properties and Functions of Interleukin-10. *Adv. Immunol.* 56: 1–26.
9. Yssel, H. and deWaal Malefyt, R. (1994) Human T-cells and interleukin-10. *In:* J.E. deVries and R. deWaal Malefyt (eds): *Interleukin-10.* R.G. Landes Company, Austin, Texas.
10. deWaal Malefyt, R., Figdor, C.G. and deVries, J.E. (1994) Regulation of human monocyte functions by interleukin-10. *In:* J.E. deVries and R. deWaal Malefyt (eds): *Interleukin-10.* R.G. Landes Company, Austin, Texas.
11. deVries, J.E. and deWaal Malefyt, R. (1995) IL-10 is a potent immunosuppressant. *Drug News and Perspectives* 8: 84–88.
12. Narula, S.K., Smith, S.R. and Rybak, M.E. (1995) Biological Activities and Clinical Potential of Interleukin-10. *In:* R. Mertelsmann and F. Herrmann (eds): *Hematopoietic Growth Factors in Clinical Applications,* 2nd Edition, Marcel Dekker Inc. pp 295–314.
13. deVries, J.E. and deWaal Malefyt, R. (1996) Immunosuppressive and anti-inflammatory effects of human IL-10. *In:* E. Faist, A.E. Baue and F.W. Schildberg (eds): *The Immune Consequences of Trauma, Shock and Sepsis. Mechanisms And Therapeutics Approaches,* Pabst Science Publishers, Lengerich, pp 302–307.
14. Kühn, R., Lohler, J., Rennick, D., Rajewsky and K., Müller, W. (1993) Interleukin-10 deficient mice develop chronic enterocolitis. *Cell* 75: 263–274.
15. Rennick, D., Davidson, N. and Berg, D. (1995) Interleukin-10 gene knock-out mice: a model of chronic inflammation. *Clin. Immunol. Immunopathol.* 76: S174-S178.
16. Berg, D., Davidson, N., Kühn, R., Müller, W., Menon, S., Holland G., Thompson-Snipes, L., Leach, M. and Rennick, D. (1996) Enterocolitis and colon cancer in interleukin-10-deficient mice are associated with aberrant cytokine production and CD4+ Th1-like responses. *J. Clin. Invest.*; *in press.*
17. Powrie, F., Leach, M.W., Mauze, S., Barcombe Caddle, L. and Coffman, R.L. (1993) Phenotypically distinct subsets of CD4+ T-cells induce or protect from chronic intestinal inflammation in C.B-17 *scid* mice. *Int. Immunol.* 5: 1461–1471.
18. Powrie, F., Leach, M.W., Mauze, S., Menon, S., Barcomb Caddle, L. and Coffman, R.L. (1994) Inhibition of Th1 responses prevents inflammatory bowel disease in *scid* mice reconstituted with CD45RBhi CD4+ T-cells. *Immunity* 1: 553–562.
19. Herfarth, H.H., Mohanty, S., Rath, H.C. and Sartor, R.B. (1996) IL-10 therapy suppresses experimental chronic, granulomatous inflammation induced by bacterial cell wall polymers. *Gut*; *in press.*

AAS 49
Therapeutic Strategies for Modulating the Inflammatory Diseases
© 1998 Birkhäuser Verlag Basel/Switzerland

Ro 45-2081, a TNF receptor fusion protein, prevents inflammatory responses in the airways

P.R. Gater and L.M. Renzetti

Hoffmann-La Roche Inc., 340 Kingsland St, Nutley, NJ 07042, USA

Summary. The TNF receptor fusion protein, Ro 45-2081, inhibited allergic and non-allergic inflammatory responses in the airways. Treatment of sensitized guinea-pigs with Ro 45-2081 reduced allergen-induced influx of inflammatory cells into the lungs, abolished edema formation and inhibited hyperreactivity to substance P. Administration of Ro 45-2081 after allergen challenge reversed the influx of inflammatory cells into the lungs. Sephadex-induced neutrophil influx into the lungs of rats was also blocked by Ro 45-2081. The effects of Ro 45-2081 suggest that inhibitors of TNF may have potential as therapeutics for inflammatory diseases in the lung.

Introduction

Tumor necrosis factor (TNF) is an inflammatory cytokine which has been implicated in the pathophysiology of a number of lung diseases. TNF-α is produced by a number of cells in the airways, including macrophages, eosinophils, epithelial cells and mast cells, in response to a variety of stimuli [1]. Elevated levels of TNF-α have been detected in either the airways or bronchoalveolar lavage (BAL) fluid from asthmatics and subjects with ARDS [2–4]. Leukocytes and monocytes from asthmatic BAL fluid release more TNF-α than cells from normal subjects [5, 6] and inhalation of TNF-α may cause airway hyperresponsivness in non-asthmatics [7]. Ro 45-2081 is a recombinant chimeric molecule constructed from the soluble 55kD human TNF receptor extracellular domain cDNA fused to the hinge region of the heavy chain IgGl gene and expressed in eukaryotic cells [8]. This TNF receptor fusion protein is a potent antagonist of TNF *in vitro* [8, 9] and prevents LPS-induced lethality in mice [8, 10]. In the present study, Ro 45-2081 was used to determine the role of TNF in animal models of allergic lung inflammation and acute lung injury.

Materials and methods

Male guinea pigs (250 to 300 g) were sensitized to ovalbumin (OA, 10 µg + 1 mg Al(OH)$_3$ in 0.5 ml sterile saline, s.c.) on days 0 and 14. Between days 21 and 28, animals were challenged

(OA, 0.1% aerosol for 30 min) and inflammatory cell influx into the lung was quantified 24 h later. Airway microvascular leakage was measured 6 h after challenge by determining the accumulation of Evans blue dye in the distal trachea and main bronchi. In order to monitor airway hyperreactivity, increases in lung resistance (R_L) evoked by substance P ($1–10$ µg/kg, i.v.) were determined by whole body plethysmography 6 h after OA challenge [3]. To evoke lung injury, male Sprague-Dawley rats ($250–350$ g) were given Sephadex G-100 suspension (7.5 mg/kg, i.v.). Inflammatory cell influx was assessed from BAL collected 24 or 72 h later [4]. Mean $\pm$ S.E.M. were calculated for all values in each experiment. Statistical differences were determined by analysis of variance on ranked data followed by multiple comparisons testing using a Student Newman-Keuls T-test, or by Student's T-test. $p < 0.05$ was considered statistically significant.

Results

Lung inflammation in the guinea-pig

The accumulation of eosinophils, neutrophils and total cells into BAL fluid 24 h after OA challenge was significantly ($p < 0.05$) inhibited by Ro 45-2081 (1 or 3 mg/kg, i.p.). When Ro 45-2081 (3 mg/kg, i.p.) was administered immediately after OA challenge, there was a significant ($p < 0.05$) reduction in the number of eosinophils and neutrophils in the BAL fluid recovered 24 h later in comparison with vehicle-treated animals (Fig. 1). This inhibitory effect was maintained for at least 72 h after OA challenge when Ro 45-2081 (3 mg/kg, i.p.) was given daily (Fig. 1).

Six hours after OA challenge the rise in Evans blue dye content in the trachea and main bronchus, which indicates an increase in airway microvascular leakage, was attenuated ($p < 0.05$) by RO 45-2081 (1 or 3 mg/kg, Fig. 2). At the same time there was a marked increase in the airway reactivity of challenged animals to substance P relative to unchallenged, sensitized guinea pigs. RO 45-2081 (3 mg/kg) caused a significant ($p < 0.05$) rightward shift of the substance P dose-response curve with a reduction in the maximum change in R_L of about 60% (Fig. 2).

Lung injury in the Sephadex-treated rat

Twenty-four hours after Sephadex administration, Ro 45-2081 (1 and 3 mg/kg, i.p.) caused a significant ($p < 0.05$) decrease in the number of neutrophils relative to the vehicle-treated group (Fig. 3). At 72 h after Sephadex, Ro 45-2081 ($1–3$ mg/kg, i.p.) caused a significant reduction ($p < 0.05$) in the number of leukocytes in BAL fluid neutrophils but a significant increase ($p < 0.05$)

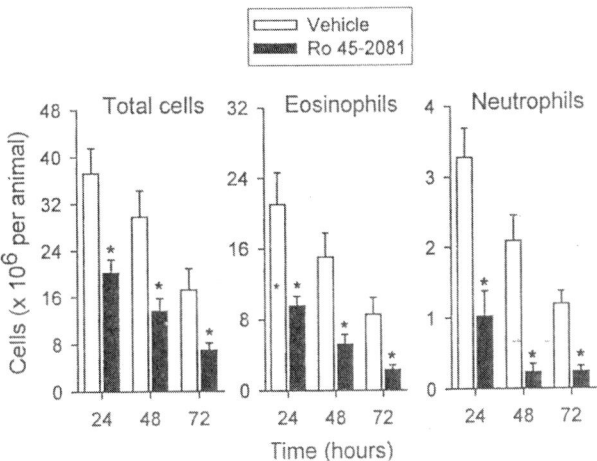

Figure 1. Reversal of OA-induced leukocyte influx into the BAL fluid of OA-challenged guiinea-pigs by Ro 45-2081 (3 mg/kg, i.p.; immediately after OA challenge and daily). Values presented are mean ± S.E.M., n=6–8, * p<0.05 relative to vehicle-treated control animals.

in the number of eosinophils. When the dose of Ro 45-2081 was increased (3 mg·kg^{-1}, i.p.), there was a significant (p<0.05) reduction in the number of total cells, macrophages, neutrophils and lymphocytes and the eosinophil count was the same as that in the vehicle-treated group.

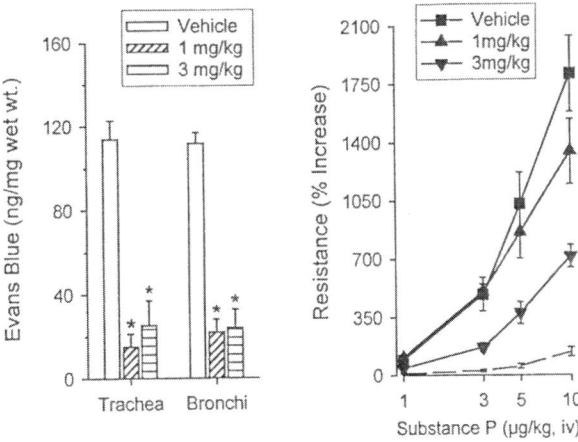

Figure 2. Inhibition of airway microvascular leakage and hyperreactivity in the guinea-pig by RO 45-2081 (1–3 mg/kg, i.p.). The dose-response curve for substance P-induced bronchoconstriction in unchallenged guinea-pigs is represented by the dashed line. Values presented are mean ± S.E.M., n=5–7, * p<0.05 relative to vehicle-treated animals.

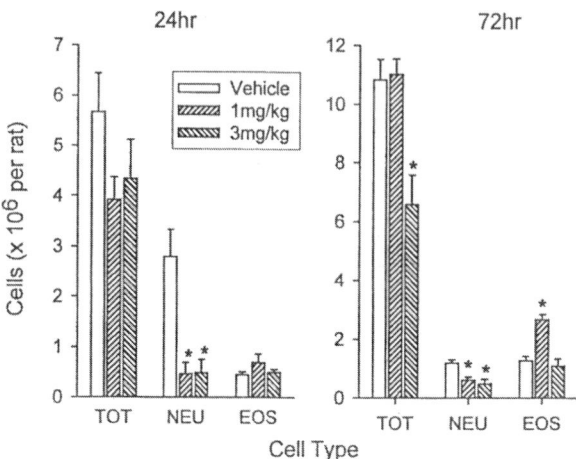

Figure 3. Inhibition of neutrophil influx into the BAL fluid of Sephadex-treated rats. Rats received Ro 45-2081 (1 or 3 mg/kg, i.p.) 1 h before administration of Sephadex (7.5 mg/kg, i.v.) and lungs were lavaged 24 h later. Values presented are mean ± S.E.M., n = 4–7, * p < 0.05 relative to vehicle-treated control animals.

Conclusion

The TNF receptor fusion protein, Ro 45-2081, caused a marked reduction of responses evoked by allergic and non-allergic provocation in the lungs of guinea-pigs and rats. The greatest effects of Ro 45-2081 were seen on neutrophil infiltration into the lungs following both allergen challenge of guinea-pigs and Sephadex challenge of rats. Since Ro 45-2081 also partly inhibited the accumulation of eosinophils in antigen-challenged guinea-pigs, TNF appears to have a role as one of the mediators of leukocyte recruitment into the airways. Airway microvascular leak in the antigen-challenged guinea-pig was completely abolished by Ro 45-2081 which suggests that TNF is an important factor in the edematous component of the response. In addition, these studies have provided evidence that TNF may also contribute to allergen-induced airway hyperreactivity in sensitized guinea-pigs. The effects of Ro 45-2081 on a number of components of inflammation in the lung suggest that compounds which inhibit TNF may be useful in the treatment of a number of pulmonary diseases.

References

1. Barnes, P.J. (1994) Cytokines as mediators of chronic asthma. *Am. J. Respir. Crit. Care Med.* 150: S42–S49.
2. Ying, S., Robinson, D.S., Varney, V., Meng, Q., Tsicopoulos, A., Moqbel, R., Durham, S.R., Kay, A.B. and Hamid, Q. (1991) TNF alpha mRNA expression in allergic inflammation. *Clin. Exp. Allergy* 21: 745–750.
3. Broide, D.H., Lotz, M., Cuomo, A.J., Coburn, D.A., Federman, E.C. and Wasserman, S.I. (1992) Cytokines in symptomatic asthma airways. *J. Allergy Clin. Immunol.* 89: 958–967.
4. Suter, P.M., Suter, S., Girardin, E., Roux-Lombard, P., Grau, G.E. and Dayer, J.-M. (1992) High bronchoalveolar levels of tumor necrosis factor and its inhibitors, interleukin-1, interferon, and elastase in patients with adult respiratory distress syndrome after trauma, shock, or sepsis. *Am. Rev. Respir. Dis.* 145: 1016–1022.
5. Cembrzynska-Nowak, M., Szklarz, E., Inglot, A.D. and Teodorczyk-Injeyan, J.A. (1993) Elevated release of tumor necrosis factor-alpha and interferon-gamma by bronchoalveolar leukocytes from patients with bronchial asthma. *Am. Rev. Respir. Dis.* 147: 291–295.
6. Gosset, P., Tsicopoulos, A., Wallaert, B., Vannimenus, C., Joseph, M., Tonnel, A.-B. and Capron, A. (1991) Increased secretion of tumor necrosis factor-α and interleukin-6 by alveolar macrophages consecutive to the development of the late asthmatic reaction. *J. Allergy Clin. Immunol.* 8: 561–571.
7. Thomas P,.S., Yates, D.H. and Barnes, P.J. (1995) Tumor necrosis factor-α increases airway responsiveness and sputum neutrophilia in normal human subjects. *Am. J. Respir. Crit. Care. Med.* 152: 76–80.
8. Ashkenazi, A., Marsters, S.A., Capon, D.J., Chamow, S.M., Figari, I.S., Pennica, D., Goeddel, D.V., Palladino, M.A. and Smith, D.H. (1991) Protection against endotoxic shock by a tumor necrosis factor receptor immunoadhesin. *Proc. Natl. Acad. Sci. USA* 88: 10535–10539.
9. Loetscher, H., Grentz, R., Zulauf, M., Lustig, A., Tabuchi, H., Schlaerger, E.J., Brockhaus, M., Gallati, H., Manneberg, M. and Lesslauer, W. (1991) Recombinant 55-kDa tumor necrosis factor receptor: Stoichiometry of binding to TNFα and TNFβ and inhibition of TNF activity. *J. Biol. Chem.* 266: 18324–18329.
10. Lesslauer, W., Tabuchi, H., Reiner, G., Brockhaus, M., Sclaeger, E.J., Grau, G., Piguet, P.F., Poitaire, P., Vassalli, P. and Loetscher, H. (1991) Recombinant soluble tumor necrosis facter receptor proteins protect mice from lipopolysaccharide-induced lethality. *Eur. J. Immunol.* 21: 2883–2886.

Summaries of workshops and poster discussions

Coordinators:

Lisa A. Marshall (SmithKline Beecham)
James D. Winkler (SmithKline Beecham)

AAS 49
Therapeutic Strategies for Modulating the Inflammatory Diseases
© 1998 Birkhäuser Verlag Basel/Switzerland

Pulmonary inflammation

C.R. Turner (Pfizer) and C.W Scott (Zenica)

This session covered a broad range of topics within the field of pulmonary inflammation. For purposes of presentation and discussion, studies were grouped into one of three subheadings: 1) eosinophil-related studies, 2) novel anti-inflammatory therapies and 3) models to examine inflammatory processes.

Watson et al. administered IL-13 (1–100 ng) intratracheally prior to antigen challenge or before instillation of TNF-α. Both TNF-α and antigen caused a significant increase (approximately 20-fold) in eosinophils, and this was significantly abrogated by IL-13, suggesting that IL-13 may modulate pulmonary inflammation. This effect is somewhat surprising given that IL-4, which shares many biological actions with IL-13, is known to enhance airway eosinophilia in mice. The role of another biochemical mediator, RANTES, was evaluated by Campbell et al. The activity of guinea pig (cloned from ConA-stimulated spleen cells, expressed in *E. coli*) and human RANTES were compared. Both induced the migration of human blood eosinophils, but not guinea pig peritoneal eosinophils. However, guinea pig peritoneal macrophages were activated *in vitro* by guinea pig RANTES as measured by an increase in intracellular calcium. In addition, tracheal instillation of the chemokine induced an increase in BAL macrophage number. The authors concluded that the guinea pig demonstrates novel cellular selectivity which may have a bearing on inflammatory responses of this model. The third presentation in this section was by Stelts et al. who administered a NOS inhibitor (L-NAME) 0.5 h prior to, and 4 h after ovalbumin (OA) challenge in sensitized mice. L-NAME significantly reduced the number of eosinophils after OA whereas D-NAME had no effect. OA-induced eosinophilia was restored if mice were co-administered excess NOS substrate plus L-NAME. Because mRNA and iNOS protein were not increased in the lungs after OA, the authors concluded that although NO contributes to the development of pulmonary eosinophilia, the iNOS form of the enzyme is not involved.

In the novel therapy section, Sehring et al. evaluated the new inhaled corticosteroid, mometasone furoate (MF), a compound with low oral absorption that lessens the potential risks associated with systemic exposure. Mice were administered MF by MDI actuation into an exposure chamber (dose range: 0.5–33 µk/kg) 24, 18 and 2 h prior to OA challenge. MF treatment reduced pulmonary eosinophil number and also the number of Thy1[+,] Th cells and the percentage of CD44[+] Th cells. IL-4, IL-5 and IFN-γ mRNA were also lower in MF-treated mice. In their poster, Kudlacz et al. (presented by RW Knippenberg) demonstrated that the combined NK-1/NK-2 antagonist, MDL 105, 172 A, reduced SP-induced inositol phosphate production *in vitro*. It also inhibited SP-induced microvascular leakage and β-Ala^8 NKA 4–10 bronchoconstriction in guinea pigs. MDL 105, 172 A also reduced capsaicin-induced dyspnea and cough. In their study, Selig et al. demonstrated that in rats administered human neutrophil elastase, a significant increase in the number of lung erythrocytes was observed 2 h post insult. Treatment with elastase inhibitors, including CE-2072, dose-dependently reduced lung hemorrhage in the rat model.

In the final section, O'Brien et al. induced plasma extravasation by administering PAF to Wistar rats that were depleted of platelets or neutrophils. They also treated rats in each group with either tranexamic acid (TXA) and aprotinin (APR), two compounds that are inhibitory in the plasminogen/plasmin pathway. The authors determined that vascular permeability was increased when either APR or TXA was administered to neutrophil-depleted rats; however, results of either drug in combination with platelet depletion were not as consistent. They concluded that neutrophils, but not platelets, may mediate the inhibitory effects of both drugs on PAF-induced plasma extravasation. Raymond et al. used a mouse model to demonstrate the protective effects of cyclosporine on pulmonary inflammation induced by respiratory syncytial virus (RSV) administered to the animals intranasally. Mice were injected with Cyclosporine one day prior to RSV innoculation and every day thereafter through day 5 and lavaged on day 6. Cyclosporine, at 100 mg/kg, completely inhibited airway inflammation, edema and necrosis. Finally, Salafia et al. compared the inflammatory responses of A/J and BALBc mice. They found that sensitized A/J mice had significantly more lavage eosinophils, serum IgE and IL-4 after OA challenge than BALBc mice. Dexamethasone treatment similarly reduced inflammatory responses in both strains, but A/J mice were much more responsive to treatment with an antibody to IL-4, 11b11. These results illustrate the necessity of complete model characterization since mechanisms underlying inflammatory responses may vary considerably depending on the model in use.

AAS 49
Therapeutic Strategies for Modulating the Inflammatory Diseases
© 1998 Birkhäuser Verlag Basel/Switzerland

New drugs for inflammatory diseases

J. Evans (Merck Frosst) and K. Tramposch (Bristol-Myers Squibb)

This workshop of eight presentations profiled inhibitors and antagonists of pro-inflammatory mediators such as LTB_4, PGE_2 and PAF. The workshop was divided into disease targets, beginning with inflammatory bowel disease (IBD), followed by new generation NSAIDs targeting arthritic diseases and ending with allergic and respiratory disease targets. The general theme of the presentations stressed improved selectivity of compounds against specific targets and improved safety profiles by a number of different strategies. W. Smith (Searle) profiled SC-57461, a potent, selective LTA_4 hydrolase inhibitor which was effective in the colitic cotton top tamarin (CTT) model. This compound blocks LTA_4 hydrolase activity *in vitro* with an IC_{50} of 23 nM. When given orally to CTT (10 mg/kg, BID), the level of LTB_4 in rectal dialysate was reduced by 90 %. It remains to be seen if a selective LTA_4 hydrolase inhibitor would confer any advantage in IBD over a leukotriene synthesis inhibitor such as MK-0591 which has not shown significant efficacy in spite of excellent inhibition of LTB_4 synthesis. One unknown factor with the selective LTA_4 hydrolase inhibitor is whether its inhibition of the aminopeptidase activity of the enzyme could have beneficial effect. Since the natural peptide substrate for this activity is unknown this cannot be predicted. Four presentations emphasized the inhibition of pro-inflammatory prostaglandins including two dual cyclooxygenase/5-lipoxygenase inhibitors. A number of questions were posed to each of these speakers as to the degree of safety offered by each type of compound. D. Kellstein (Proctor and Gamble) reviewed the preclinical profile of PGV-20229. This compound is a dual inhibitor of cyclooxygenase (COX) and 5-lipoxygenase (5-LO) with a 100-fold selectivity for COX-2. This compound had analgesic activity in the mouse phenylquinone writhing assay comparable to naproxen (~1 mg/kg). G.I. safety was evaluated in rats and dogs. No lesions were observed in dogs given PGV-20229 orally (25 mg/kg/day) for 5 days. It is not known at this time what contribution the lipoxygenase inhibitory properties of this compound has to the overall G.I. safety profile. R. Dyer (Parke-Davis) described the pharmacology of CI-1004. This compound is equally potent against 5-LO and COX-2 (IC_{50} ~400 nM). It does not appear to be active against COX-1. This compound demonstrates anti-arthritic activity in animals without inducing toxicity in chronic dosing (up to 13 weeks). E. Grimm (Merck Frosst) described a new class of selective COX-2 inhibitors. These compounds were classified as 5, 5-disubstituted 3, 4-diaryl-2-(5H)-furanone methylsulfones and showed 20–300-fold selectivity for COX-

2 vs COX-1. These compounds had analgesic activity with no gastric side-effects. G. Cirino (University of Naples) described a different approach toward reducing G.I. irritation. HCT-3012 is a nitroxybutylester of naproxen which is designed to release a nitrate moiety. *In vivo* this compound had activity comparable to naproxen (~1 mg/kg) in analgesia models but did not cause G.I. damage at ~100 mg/kg. Questions were poised concerning the degree of ester cleavage of this "prodrug" and the potential for induction of tolerance to the released nitrate. It remains to be seen in clinic which of these approaches will offer the most effective therapy against arthritic pain and inflammation. The workshop ended with three presentations targeting allergic and asthmatic diseases. D. Albert (Abbott Labs) demonstrated that the potent and selective PAF antagonist ABT-491 inhibited nasal vascular permeability associated with experimental allergic rhinitis in Brown Norway rats. E. Walker (Zeneca) profiled ZD-4407 a potent, selective, non-redox inhibitor of 5-lipoxygenase that evolved from a methyl derivative of ZD-2318. The methyl derivative methoxytetrahydropyrans are more potent *in vivo* than the non-methylated equivalent compounds due to lack of autoinduction of their own metabolism. ZD-2318 and ZD-4407 are no longer in clinical development due to Zeneca's choice of the cysLT1 (LTD$_4$ antagonist Accolate™ as their key anti-leukotriene anti-asthmatic therapy). R. Harris (Abbott Labs) gave the final talk of this workshop on the development of a new series of leukotriene biosynthesis inhibitors with 5-LO-activating protein (FLAP) as their target. He described the development of iminocarboxylate FLAP inhibitors and the profile of the potent, orally active enantiomer A-93178. This compound was active *in vitro versus* human whole blood LTB$_4$ formation (IC$_{50}$ ~870 nM) and *in vivo* in bronchoconstrictive and inflammatory models, but had the drawbacks of a difficult enantioselective synthesis and a short-half life in the monkey.

AAS 49
Therapeutic Strategies for Modulating the Inflammatory Diseases
© 1998 Birkhäuser Verlag Basel/Switzerland

Cartilage and bone

W.V. Williams (University of Pennsylvania) and J. Rediske (CIBA)

The Cartilage and Bone session was introduced by John Rediske. He pointed out that there were two main thrusts in the presentations: investigation of mediators/process involved in tissue degradation, specifically cellular enzymes, using novel compounds; and newer mediators which may retard tissue damage, such as IL-4, or play a pathogenic role, such as fibronectin fragments.

M.J. Janusz presented studies of the human neutrophil elastase inhibitor MDL 101, 146 in two experimental models of inflammatory arthritis: collagen induced arthritis (CIA) and adjuvant arthritis (AA). DA rats were immunized with bovine type II collagen on day 0, dosed with MDL 101, 146 on day 10 (250 mg/kg/day), and evaluated for joint swelling and later for chondro-protection. There was a mild but statistically significant reduction of tibio-tarsal joint swelling in the treated rats. On histological examination, there was marked diminution of cartilage destruction and pannus formation with the drug, while bone destruction was essentially unaffected. Similar but less marked changes were seen in the intertarsal points. In contrast, the drug had virtually no effect in the AA model. These data suggest that cartilage destruction in CIA is at least partially dependent on neutrophil elastase, and indicate that the choice of model system plays a significant role in determining the potential efficacy of novel therapies.

R.C. Borghaei presented *in vitro* studies of interleukin-4 (IL-4) regulation of matrix metallo-proteinases (MMPs) production by synovial fibroblasts. She noted that IL-1, which is increased in the synovial fluid of patients with rheumatoid arthritis (RA), has been linked to the induction of increased levels of MMP-1 (collagenase) and MMP-3 (stromelysin) by synovial fibroblasts. In contrast, the "anti-inflammatory" cytokine IL-4 is virtually undetectable in RA synovial fluid. They observed that MMP-1 and MMP-3 mRNA levels in RA synovial fibroblasts increased following addition of IL-1, and that IL-4 markedly diminished MMP mRNA levels in this system to ~30–40% of control levels, with an IC50 of 0.3 ng/mL. Additional studies with reporter gene constructs using the MMP-3 promoter confirmed these results. She concluded that cytokine imbalance in RA may be important in the development of joint destruction.

R. Goldberg presented *in vivo* studies on the matrix metalloproteinase (MMP) inhibitor CGS27023 A. CGS27023 A is an orally active synthetic MMP with nM potency against stro-myelysin, collagenase and gelatinase. The effect of this compound on cartilage proteoglycan was examined in an experimental rabbit model of OA in which joint pathology was initiated by

surgical removal of the lateral meniscus (MNX). They found minimal cartilage matrix degradation, as measured by the ratio of glycosaminoglycans to hydroxyproline, between weeks 4–16
and significant matrix loss by 20 weeks post MNX. Appearance of the cartilage proteoglycan
3B3(-) epitope, a marker of cartilage repair which appears on newly synthesized proteoglycan,
exhibited a steady increase from wk 4 to 12 and sharply declined to initial levels by week 20.
Therapeutic treatment of rabbits with 100 mg/kg CGS27023 A from day 8 to 20 resulted in maintenance of proteoglycan content at levels equivalent to control and an approximately 3 fold
increase in 3B3(-) cartilage epitope compared to MNX control groups. These studies implicate
matrix metalloproteinases as key mediators of cartilage degradation in this experimental model of
OA and suggest that inhibitors of this class of enzyme would retard cartilage destruction and
facilitate repair of the matrix in OA.

F. J. van de Loo presented some intriguing findings on the role of IL-6 and nitric oxide on IL-
1-mediated joint pathology using two knock-out strains:1) IL-6 and 2) iNOs. The experimental
model used for these studies was an intra-articular IL-1 injection model in which IL-1 causes a
depression of proteoglycan (PG) synthesis followed by enhanced PG synthesis (recovery phase)
at 5 days post IL-1. They first examined the effects of IL-1 on cartilage proteoglycan synthesis in
an IL-6 knock-out mouse strain and found that IL-1 suppressed proteoglycan synthesis about
50% in the IL-6 knock-out strain and normal control animals. Additionally, there was a trend that
cartilage from the IL-6 knock-out mice exhibited a decreased recovery response to IL-1. In contrast, IL-1-stimulated suppression of proteoglycan synthesis and corresponding proteoglycan
synthesis recovery phase was completely blocked in the iNOs knock-out mice compared to normal control animals. Finally, they showed that the depressed proteoglycan synthesis response to
IGF-1 in IL-1-treated cartilage was also dependent on nitric oxide. These data suggest that IL-1
induced NO plays a key role in IL-1-mediated suppression of proteoglycan synthesis while IL-6
may promote the recovery phase of cartilage proteoglycan synthesis.

C.J. Dunn and colleagues examined the effect of diphosphonates (DP), which have been used
therapeutically for osteoporosis and other diseases associated with loss of bone, in models of
acute and chronic inflammation. Compounds used included dichloromethylene diphosphonic acid
and more novel structures. They found that oral dosing with DP's had no effect on carageenan
pleurisy or the reverse passive arthus reaction in rats. These compounds, however, suppressed a
DTH granuloma response in mice. Additionally, DP's showed disease modifying activity in three
models of arthritis (BSA-induced, adjuvant-induced, and collagen II-induced) characterized by
significant protection of bone and cartilage resorption. While there was little evidence for DP's
affecting the immune response, this class of compounds appeared to affect monocyte-macro-
phage development/function *in vivo*. The anti-inflammatory mechanisms of these compounds remains unknown. These results suggest that diphosphonates, in addition to affecting bone turn-

over, have anti-inflammatory properties and may provide a novel two hit (bone and tissue injury) therapeutic approach for rheumatoid arthritis.

E. C. Arner described the *in vivo* effects of fibronectin fragments on *in vivo* cartilage metabolism and inflammation. In previous studies, Arner and colleagues described the ability of fibronectin fragments to induce cartilage breakdown and matrix metalloproteinase (MMP) production by isolated rabbit chondrocytes. In this study, they examined the *in vivo* activities of these fibronectin fragments in an intra-articular injection model in the rabbit. They found that injection of 2 mg synthetic RGD peptide induced an increase in cell influx and proteoglycosaminoglycan (PG) release into the synovial fluid, increased synovial levels of MMP, and minimal changes in cartilage PG synthesis and content. Injection of 1 μM of the fibronectin proteolytic fragment fn120, containing the RGD attachment site, caused a more dramatic cell influx, MMP, and PG response. Importantly, this fragment also caused a decrease in cartilage proteoglycan synthesis and content. These results suggest a possible role for extracellular matrix-integrin interactions as regulators of cartilage turnover in arthritis.

Some final thoughts... The general discussion was initiated by Sonya Shortkoff, who observed that antigen induced arthritis has a chronic irreversible phase. Similar observations are present in human rheumatoid arthritis. This clearly presents a challenge to therapeutic development. Have modulators/inhibitors been tried in the chronic phases of these disease models? What do we even know about pathogenesis?

It was postulated that perhaps fibronectin (FN) fragments (mentioned by Dr. Arner to be present in human arthritis in μM amounts, effective in her system to induce cell influx and proteoglycan/cartilage degradation) are generated and develop into a positive feedback loop. They may induce MMPs and other proteases which degrade proteoglycans. PGs are notable for their "slipperiness" (cells do not stick to them) while FN fragments generated induce cellular influx. This may lead to chronicity. The loop might be:

Initial damage → FN fragment generation → MMP induction → perpetuation of damage → PG degradation → FN deposition → more MMP induction → etc.

The system is complex, as multiple cell populations and signals are involved. The example of CIA in rats was given. When induced by immunization *in vivo*, destructive arthritis results. Active disease can't be transferred by T-cells alone or antibody alone, both are needed for disease induction. Regulation of the inflammatory response also may be complex. The point was made that in acute arthritis (eg. gout), the same initial insults are there, but what limits disease and prevents chronicity is unknown. Could cytokines such as IL-4 be produced to down modulate disease?

Clearly more studies need to be done to better understand the cellular and molecular basis for acute and chronic arthritis. We all should have jobs for years to come!

Transcriptional regulation and inflammation

T. Leff (Parke-Davis) and V.J. Palombella (ProScript)

Transcription factors play a central role in the immune and inflammatory response. Transcriptional regulators such as NF-κB (p50/p65), AP-1 (c-fos/c-jun), IRF-1, and nuclear hormone receptors can either stimulate or repress the gene expression of a number of pro-inflammatory mediators including cytokines, chemokines and cell adhesion molecules. Importantly, the activity of these transcription factors is regulated *via* an elaborate series of intracellular signal transduction events in response to extracellular stimuli. This workshop emphasized the complex role of various transcription factors in inflammation and addressed some of the signaling events involved in their regulation. Methods to control the activity of particular transcription factors was also highlighted during the presentations. A brief summary of the six papers presented at the "Transcriptional Modulation" workshop are described below.

While many pro-inflammatory signals exert influence on gene expression indirectly *via* intracellular signaling cascades initiated by cell surface receptors, some signaling molecules may act directly on transcriptional activity of target genes through the action of a class of transcription factors called nuclear receptors. This large and diverse family of proteins are ligand activated transcription factors that include the steroid hormone receptors, the vitamin D and retinoic acid receptors and a large number orphan receptors for which ligands have not been identified. Dr. Irmgard Wiesenberg (Ciba-Geigy) presented evidence indicating that a class of anti-arthritic thiazolidinediones can bind with high affinity to a nuclear receptor called RZR/RORα. In addition, results from cell based transcription assays clearly demonstrated that these compounds are specific and potent activators of RZR/RORα dependent transcription. Finally, comparison of structurally related compounds showed a direct correlation between receptor binding activity and anti-arthritic activity. Dr. Wiesenberg proposed that the anti-arthritic effects of these compounds may be explained by regulation of specific (as yet unidentified) immuno-modulatory genes by an RZR/RORα dependent mechanism. An interesting and potentially significant aspect of this work is the recent proposal that the pineal gland hormone melatonin is an endogenous ligand for the RZR/RORα receptor.

The intracellular effects inflammatory cytokines are thought to be mediated, at least in part, by MAPK (mitogen activated protein kinase) signaling pathways. One of the important components of this complex signaling network (especially with regard to transcriptional regulation) is the

MAPK homolog called Jnk (c-Jun N-terminal kinase). This protein kinase increases the activity of the transcription factor c-Jun (and probably many others) by serine phosphorylation. Although multiple Jnk isoforms have been identified, very little is known of their specific activities and cellular effects. Dr. Wendi Feeser (DuPont/Merck) presented a paper characterizing the recently identified Jnk isoform, Jnk1b, and comparing its activity the standard Jnk1 isoform. These two isoforms are identical accept for 8 amino acid substitutions in the kinase domains IX and X. Both enzymes were found to be expressed in the same cell-types and to be phosphorylated by the same upstream protein kinase (MKK4). In addition both enzymes appeared to respond to the same set of stimuli in transfected cells. There were, however, some measurable differences in the enzymatic activities of the two isoforms. The Jnk1b isoform showed a higher basal activity and had a slightly higher affinity for the substrate c-Jun. These differences may reflect distinct functional roles for the Jnk1 and Jnk1b isoforms.

Many genes that are activated by inflammatory signals are transcriptionally regulated by either AP-1 (c-Jun/c-Fos dimers) or by NF-κB or both. Glucocorticoid hormones, acting through the glucocorticoid receptor (GR), have been shown to repress the transcriptional activity of AP-1 and NF-κB dependent genes. Dr. Evelyne Delorme (Ligand) presented the results from experiments designed to characterize the mechanistic relationship between the repression of AP-1 activity and the repression of NF-κB activity by glucocorticoids. The role of the DNA binding domain of the GR was examined by using a GR containing a mutation in one of the zinc fingers required for DNA binding. The ability of wild-type and mutant GR to repress transcription from natural and artificial promoters regulated by either AP-1 alone, NF-κB alone or by both transcription factors was examined. In transient transfection assays, the effect of ligand activated wild-type and mutant GR on transcription from AP-1 dependent *vs.* NF-κB dependent promoters was significantly different. These results suggest that ligand activated GR may influence AP-1 dependent transcriptional activity and NF-κB dependent transcriptional activity by distinct mechanisms. A possible explanation for these results is that AP-1 and NF-kB proteins interact with distinct sites on the GR.

IL-1β is a very important pro-inflammatory cytokine and understanding the many mechanisms by which it promotes the inflammatory response is crucial. To this end, the regulation of IL-1β induced PGE_2 production by NF-κB was discussed by Amy Roshak (Smith Kline). IL-1β stimulates the formation of prostaglandin E_2 (PGE_2) in human rheumatoid synovial fibroblasts (RSF). IL-1β also induces the expression of 85 kDa-phospholipase A_2 (PLA_2) and the inducible form of cyclooxygenase (COX-2) in these cells. Since both these enzymes are required for PGE_2 production, it appears as though IL-1β is increasing PGE_2 production *via* the increased expression of these two enzymes. An analysis of the promoter regions of both the 85 kDa-PLA_2 and COX-2 genes has identified potential NF-κB consensus binding sites. In addition, gel shift analysis identified a p65 containing NF-κB DNA binding complex in nuclear extracts from IL-1β stimulated RSF. Importantly, antisense oligonucleotide and consensus oligonucleotide decoy experiments indicated that the p65 subunit of NF-κB is required for IL-1β induced PGE_2 formation and the IL-1β inducible expression of the 85 kDa-PLA_2 and COX-2 genes. Interestingly, antisense oligonucleotides directed against p50 or c-rel had no effect on PGE_2 production by RSF. These data provide direct evidence for the requirement of p65/NF-κB in stimulating both COX-2 and 85 kDa-PLA_2 inducible gene expression and the participation of NF-κB in prostanoid formation in RSF. These results extend the list of pro-inflammatory mediators regulated by NF-κB and strengthen the role for NF-κB as a key regulator of the inflammatory response.

Ruth Thornton (Philadelphia College of Osteopathic Medicine) presented a paper on the interplay between inflammatory cytokines, namely IL-1β, and the molecular response to hypoxic conditions. This presentation again illustrated the complexity of the cellular responses to pro-inflammatory cytokines. Dr. Thornton discussed the possible connection between IL-1 in rheumatoid arthritis (RA) and hypoxic conditions that may arise in the joints of RA patients. The connection between IL-1 and hypoxia lies in the fact that IL-1 stimulates the DNA binding activity of Hypoxia Inducible Factor-1 (HIF-1) in synovial and gingival fibroblasts. HIF-1 is a heterodimeric transcription factor (α/β). HIF-1β is constitutively expressed, while HIF-1α is inducible by hypoxia or $CoCl_2$. HIF-1 has not been fully characterized, but it is known to activate the transcription of several glycolytic enzymes and vascular endothelial growth factor (VEGF), which could be important in RA since it promotes angiogenesis. IL-1β also induces the steady state levels of HIF-1α mRNA in synovial and gingival fibroblasts. However, this is not responsible for the increased DNA binding activity of HIF-1, since IL-1β induced the DNA binding of HIF-1 in the presence of cycloheximide. Follow up studies should clarify the connection between IL-1β or other pro-inflammatory cytokines and the cellular response to hypoxia.

Previous studies have suggested that high concentrations of aspirin can inhibit the activation of NF-κB and that this is responsible for some of aspirin's anti-inflammatory properties. However, follow up studies have also shown that these concentrations of aspirin can have effects on other transcription factors by effecting particular protein kinases. Therefore the ability of aspirin to specifically inhibit the activation of NF-κB remains a matter of debate. Along these lines, Sidney Morris (University of Pittsburgh) presented a paper demonstrating another novel effect of aspirin on the transcription factor interferon regulatory factor-1 (IRF-1). The transcription factor IRF-1 participates with NF-κB, HMG I/Y and ATF-2 in promoting the transcription of the IFN-β gene. In addition, IRF-1 has been shown to have an effect on cellular proliferation. He showed that unlike NF-κB, aspirin (3–10 mM) can stimulate the expression of IRF-1 mRNA in response to LPS or IFN-γ in a macrophage cell line. Indomethacin had no effect, indicating that this effect was specific to aspirin and not other NSAIDs. Importantly, aspirin or salicylate enhance IRF-1 expression even when added several hours after LPS treatment. This suggests that aspirin could be working post-transcriptionally or post-translationally to stabilize the IRF-1 mRNA or protein, respectively. Since IRF-1 is involved in the regulation of IFN-β gene expression, and IFN-β can modulate the inflammatory response, the results presented by Dr. Morris suggest that aspirin can also inhibit the inflammatory response by driving the expression of IFN-β. Furthermore, IRF-1 is involved in the regulation of other pro-inflammatory proteins, therefore aspirin could enhance the inflammatory response in addition to inhibiting it depending upon the response. More work is needed to identify and characterize the anti-inflammatory mechanism(s) of action of aspirin including its effects on IRF-1 biosynthesis and NF-κB activation.

In summary, the diversity of subjects presented at this workshop attests to the important role of transcriptional regulation in a wide range of inflammatory responses. In addition, the variety of transcription factors discussed suggests that transcriptional regulatory mechanisms relevant to inflammation will not be limited to a specific subset regulatory proteins or mechanisms. In any case, it is clear that many key events in the inflammation process occur at the level of gene expression, and that further exploration of transcriptional mechanisms in inflammation will provide new insights into the inflammatory process as well as novel targets for therapeutic intervention.

AAS 49
Therapeutic Strategies for Modulating the Inflammatory Diseases
© 1998 Birkhäuser Verlag Basel/Switzerland

Cytokines/apoptosis

D.J. Livingston (Vertex Pharmaceuticals)

Pro-inflammatory cytokines are critical mediators of inflammation, and therapeutic strategies to inhibit pathogenic effects of these proteins are of interest for the treatment of autoimmune and inflammatory diseases. Highly specific anti-interleukin-1 (IL-1) and anti-tumor necrosis factor (TNF) therapeutics are being evaluated in the clinic. Many questions remain concerning the precise role of these cytokines and others in diseases such as rheumatoid arthritis and osteoarthritis. For example, we would like to better understand the distinct roles of these cytokines in T-cell dependent responses *vs.* T-cell independent, monocyte/macrophage-mediated responses. We would also like to know whether their pro-inflammatory effects correlate with joint cartilage erosion. Such questions can be probed by the use of selective cytokine antagonists in well-characterized animal models of disease. In the IRA Workshop on Cytokines and Apoptosis, the effects of inhibitors of TNF, IL-1 and IGF-1 in animal models of human autoimmune and inflammatory diseases were presented.

Dr. S.A. Stimpson (Glaxo Wellcome) presented studies of the role of insulin-like growth factor-1 (IGF-1) in peptidoglycan-polysaccharide (PG-PS)-induced arthritis in rats. IGF-1 levels are increased in synovial fluid of diseased joints in rheumatoid and osteoarthritis. An IGF-1 binding protein is also produced, presumably a means of biological regulation of IGF-1 activity. Stimpson and colleagues raised high-affinity monoclonal antibodies against IGF-1, and a neutralizing antibody (MAb 35I17) was selected for prophylactic injection in the rat arthritis model. The antibody had no effect on the acute T-cell independent phase of arthritis, but selectively inhibited the chronic, T-cell dependent fibrotic and erosive phase. MAb 35I17 was capable of suppressing free IGF-1 in the serum in five of nine rats, while the other animals in the cohort showed evidence of an antiidiotypic response. Animals with lowered levels of IGF-1 were protected in this model, with the readouts being granulatoma, histopathological evaluation of joints, and pyridinium cross-link release. Pyridinium cross links detected in the urine of diseased animals correlated with matrix destruction in the joints.

Three reports concerned strategies to reduce TNF activity *in vivo,* using either synthetic inhibitors of TNF-α production or anti-TNF antibodies. Dr. B.E. Miller (Rhone-Poulenc Rorer) presented work on the regulation of TNF-α production by adenosine receptors. An endotoxin (LPS)-induced sepsis model was used in this study. Mixed A_1/A_2 receptor agonists such as

CPCA (5'-(N-cyclopropyl)-carboxamidoadenosine) administered subcutaneously 2 h prior to sensitization, suppressed LPS-induced TNF-α production. CPCA was also able to inhibit paw swelling in Streptococcal cell wall-induced arthritis in rats at doses of 30 μg/kg, although no data on chrondroprotection were presented. The A_2 receptor antagonist DMPX (3, 7-dimethyl-1-propargylxanthine), a partially selective adenosine receptor antagonist, restored production of TNF-α. Structure-activity data from a series of adenosine receptor agonists and antagonists suggested that inhibition of TNF-α production is mediated by the A2b receptor.

B.D. Jaffe (DuPont Merck) reported characterization of the immune response in rodents treated with TNF inhibitors. The inhibitors used were an anti-TNF antibody or a hydroxamate inhibitor of TNF production BB-16 (British Biotech). Testing of these agents in carrageenan- or TPA-induced edema acute models demonstrated anti-inflammatory effects. A delayed-type hypersensitivity model was chosen for discrimination between anti-inflammatory and immune suppression effects. Immune modulators are effective in the sensitization phase of the DTH model, but not in the challenge phase. The TNF inhibitors demonstrated no effect in the sensitization phase. Finally, the effect of these inhibitors on the ability of mice to elicit IgM and IgG responses to sheep red blood cells was determined. The inhibitors did not block these antibody responses, supporting the hypothesis that TNF blockade should not lead to immunosuppression. M.A. Gallo reported experiments to evaluate anti-TNF antibody (cA2, Centocor) in transgenic mice constitutively expressing TNF-α. Arthritic severity was scored after 5 weeks of intraperitoneal administration of antibody. A reduction in arthritic index of inflammation was noted in treated animals. Additionally, histological evaluation of joints showed protection by cA2 of joint architecture, and inhibition of pannus formation and synovitis.

Two papers concerned protective effects of IL-1 blockade. K.M. Gillooly presented a study in the mouse type II collagen-induced arthritis model, using the anti-IL-1 type I receptor antibody Ro25-3048 (Hoffman-LaRoche). The incidence and severity of inflammation in antibody-treated animals was significantly lower than in the control group. Notably, cessation of antibody treatment did not produce flare or sustained increases in inflammation over a period of several weeks. Additionally, Dr. Gillooly and colleagues evaluated arthritis in transgenic mice with a disrupted IL-1 receptor (Type I) gene. These animals were first back crossed into a genetic background (DBA-1/J) that are particularly susceptible to polyarthritis induced by immunogens. Modulation of LPS-induced IL-6 and TNF production was observed in the IL-1R knockout mice. These animals were also less susceptible to collagen-induced arthritis. F. van de Loo (Univ. Hosp. Nijmegen, The Netherlands) reported gene transfer of a retroviral vector encoding IL-1 receptor antagonist (C.A. Evans, University of Pittsburgh) to NIH-3 T3 cells. Injection of the transfected cells expressing IL-1RA into the right knee of DBA-1/J mice protected these animals from development of collagen-induced arthritis. Twenty-three of 29 treated animals showed no sign of polyarthritis under conditions where 17 of 20 animals in the control group developed arthritis. Examination of histology sections indicated that the anti-inflammatory effects of gene transfer correlated with protection of cartilage from destruction and synovitis.

A final presentation addressed the involvement of the interleukin-1 converting enzyme (ICE)/CPP32 family proteases (the caspases) in the apoptotic response, which occurs in synovial and immune cells of arthritic joints and in a variety of other tissues in human inflammatory diseases. J.D. Winkler (SmithKline Beecham) discussed the role of inappropriate apoptosis in varied diseases including myelodysplastic syndrome, polycystic kidney disease and osteoporosis. The caspases hydrolyze intracellular protein substrates at Asp-X sequences during apoptosis. Winkler described the effects of caspase inhibitors on camptothecin-induced apoptosis of HL60 cells (a leukemic monocytic cell line) in culture. This agent stimulated the proteolytic activity of one subfamily of caspases (the CPP32-like homologs), without upregulating activity of the ICE subfamily, suggesting the principal involvement of the former in apoptosis. A caspase inhibitor was capable of blocking HL-60 apoptosis, suggesting therapeutic potential of this class of inhibitors. It is notable that dysregulation of pro-inflammatory cytokines is one of the signals that can stimulate apoptosis in pathological settings.

Therapeutic Strategies for Modulating the Inflammatory Diseases
© 1998 Birkhäuser Verlag Basel/Switzerland

New technologies and rational drug design

J.S. Skotnicki (Wyeth-Ayerst) and R.S. Jacobs (U.C.S.B)

J.G. Mohanty and coworkers (Allegheny University of the Health Sciences, Philadelphia) reported on the development of a fluorescent micro-assay of H_2O_2 release from activated eosinophils.
This assay uses N-acetyl-3, 7-dihydroxyphenoxazine (A6550) as a substrate for horseradish peroxidase (HRP). This substrate becomes highly fluorescent upon oxidation and was found to be
more stable with a linear dose response when the A6550:H_2O_2 ratio was greater than 5. The sensitivity of the assay was reported to be as low as 2 picomoles H_2O_2. A6550 was found to be at
least 10 fold higher in sensitivity than scopoletin as a substrate for horseradish peroxidase.

R.P. Carlson and co-workers (Abbott) provided results of an extensive study using micro-
scopic magnetic resonance imaging (MRI) to investigate and quantify pathological changes in the
arthritic joints of mice and rats undergoing lipopolysaccharide (LPS) potentiated Type II collagen
induced arthritis (CIA) and established adjuvant arthritis (EAA). In this study, they were able to
distinguish between mouse CIA and rat EAA histopathological changes throughout the progression of the disease without euthanizing the animals. The results using a variety of orally active
anti-inflammatory drugs were summarized.

L. Chen and coworkers (Hoffmann-LaRoche) described their efforts directed toward the
design and synthesis of a series of analogs as potential IL-2 receptor α (IL-2Rα) antagonists.
Following SAR analyses, Ro 26-4550 (N-(3-[1-aminoiminomethyl]-piperidine)acetyl-4-phenyl-
ethynylphenylalanine methyl ester was identified as a reversible, competitive IL-2 inhibitor
($IC_{50} = 3$ μM). From SAR and molecular modeling studies, a pharmacophore model was constructed suggesting that Ro 26-4550 is bound to IL-2 rather than IL-2Rα; this hypothesis was
confirmed by solution NMR perturbation experiments using ^{15}N-IL-2.

Ro 26-4550

N. Ouimet and coworkers (Merck Frosst) discussed the rationale for the design of selective cyclooxygenase-2 (Cox-2) inhibitors and summarized their work in the "sulide" class of molecules. Following SAR studies, the 4-ethylthiazole derivative L-758, 115 emerged as the best compound in this series: $IC_{50} = 6$ nM against Cox-2 and inactive in the Cox-1 assay (at 10 µM); $ED_{30} = 0.16$ mg/kg/po in the rat paw edema assay.

L-758,115

M. Russel and coworkers (Searle) summarized the SAR of a series of leukotriene A_4 hydrolase (LTA$_4$-H) inhibitors. The genesis of these efforts was SC-27716 (1-[2-[4-(phenyl)phenoxy]ethyl]pyrollidine) which was identifed by random screening of the corporate compound library. Based on this compound, rational design and synthesis furnished SC-57461 A (3-[methyl-[3-[4-(phenylmethyl)phenoxy]propyl]amino]propionic acid hydrochloride) and SC-56938 (ethyl 1-[2-[4-(phenylmethyl)phenoxy]ethyl-3-piperidinecarboxylate): $IC_{50} = 2.5$ and 40 nM, respectively.

SC-27716

SC-56938   **SC-57461A**

P.E. Finke and coworkers (Merck) reported results of an extensive study of orally active intracellular inhibitors of human leukocyte elastase (HLE). Synthesis of ethanolamine pro-drugs resulted in compounds with increased potency as determined by a whole blood HLE assay. Ethylenediamine amides proved to be metabolically stable alkaline analogs. The analog L-694, 458

([2S, 1 (1R)]-2-[4-[[(4-methyl)piperazin-1-yl]carbonyl]phenoxy]-3, 3-diethyl-N-[1-(3, 4-methylenedioxyphenyl)butyl]-4-oxo-1-azetidinecarboxamide) was found to be a selective, orally active HLE inhibitor.

L-694,458

AAS 49
Therapeutic Strategies for Modulating the Inflammatory Diseases
© 1998 Birkhäuser Verlag Basel/Switzerland

Chemokines

M.S. Barnette (SmithKline Beecham) and R. Schleimer (Johns Hopkins)

The subject of this workshop was the role that the emerging families of proteins, know as the chemokines, plays in the development and maintenance of an inflammatory reaction. Chemokines are classified into three families based on sequence homology and function. The CXC family comprises those chemokines in which the initial pair of cysteine residues are separated by a single amino acid. These proteins primarily recruit and activate neutrophils. IL-8 and Gro-α are examples of CXC chemokines. In the CC family of proteins, the initial cysteine residues are adjacent and these proteins had been shown to recruit and activate mononuclear cells, eosinophils and basophils with little or no effect on neutrophils. RANTES, MIP-1α, and MCP-1 are examples of CC chemokines. The last family to be described was the C family, of which is there only one example, lymphotactin. Lymphotactin is unique among the chemokines in that it seems to recruit only T-cells. All of these protein exert most of their biological effects through activation of seven transmembrane G-protein coupled receptors.

To introduce the role of chemokines in inflammatory processes, R. Schleimer showed the localization of RANTES within the epithelium of nasal polyps and discussed the ability of the various CC chemokines to recruit and activate eosinophils. His presentation focused on the role of the chemokine receptor CCR3 in eosinophil activation and the ability of the novel chemokine MCP-4 to activate this receptor. MCP-4 is recently described chemokine whose expression has been demonstrated in lung. Furthermore, the expression of this chemokine in lung epithelial cells appears to regulated by both pro-inflammatory stimuli, such as TNF and by anti-inflammatory agents, glucocorticoids. In several epithelial cell lines TNF will increase the expression of MCP-4 and this increase can be blocked by prior treatment with glucocorticoids. With regard to the recruitment of eosinophils, Dr. Schleimer demonstrated that MCP-4 like RANTES, MCP-3 and eotaxin will produce eosinophil chemotaxis. In addition, it appears that MCP-4 like eotaxin interacts with the CCR3 receptor expressed in eosinophils since MCP-4 can inhibit eotaxin binding to these cells and both chemokines can cross desensitize each others response. Thus CCR3 presents an interesting target to block eosinophil recruitment into inflammatory sites.

Continuing the discussion of chemokine receptors, M.S. Barnette compared the distribution and pharmacological characterization of two chemokine receptors CCR1 and CCR5. Both receptors share the ability to bind RANTES; however they demonstrate different rank order affinities for the other CC chemokines. Furthermore, CCR1 and CCR5 have unique cellular distributions. CCR1 is expressed in monocytes and macrophages, with variable level of expression in basophils, eosinophils and a low level of expression in T-cells. On the other hand, CCR5 is primarily expressed in macrophages and T-cells. Indeed, the affinity of CC chemokines for CCR5 expressed in either CHO or HEK 293 is quite similar to that observed for the RANTES receptor expressed in peripheral blood T-cells suggesting that CCR5 and not CCR1 is the RANTES receptor on T-cells. More recently, it has been reported that in addition to a potential role in regulating T-cell trafficking, CCR5 also serves as a co-receptor for HIV-1 entry in cells, especially for the macrophage tropic isolates of this virus.

To continue the discussion, R.J. Jordan discussed the ability of a variety of stimuli to induce chemokine expression in human vascular smooth muscle. Both TNF and IL-1a increased the expression of both IL-8 and MCP-1; however only TNF increased the expression of RANTES. In addition, it appears that the time course for each response is different. Both MCP-1 and IL-8 expression peaks at 6 h whereas RANTES expression is greatest after 48 h. Also Dr. Jordan showed that low density lipoproteins and PGDF increased the expression of MCP-1, but not IL-8 or RANTES. Thus demonstrating that these genes are differentially regulated in vascular smooth muscle cells and each may have a potential role in the pathophysiology of atherosclerosis.

Dr. Gladue summarized the results of his work examining the role of CC chemokines in the development of an allogeneic T-cells response. Within 24 h after implantation, high levels of several chemokines, MCP-1, MIP-1α and MIP-1β were observed within the sponge. This increase was co-incident with the accumulation of neutrophils and mononuclear cells within the implant. To determine the role of MIP-1α in this response, Dr. Gladue examined the ability of neutralizing antibodies to MIP-1α to prevent the mononuclear cell influx and examined the cellular reaction in a MIP-1α knockout mouse. In both cases, there cellular response in the sponge was unchanged suggesting the MIP-1α is not essential to the recruitment of cells in this model.

Dr. Perretti presented evidence showing that MCP-1 is important in eliciting the recruitment of monocytes into the peritoneal cavity after a zymosan challenge. MCP-1 levels in peritoneal fluid increases prior to the appearance of monocytes in the cavity. This zymosan-induced increase in MCP-1 appears to result from a stimulation of resident macrophages since resting peritoneal macrophages do not express MCP-1, as detected by RT-PCR, but peritoneal macrophages from zymosan-stimulated animals, express MCP-1. Furthermore, a neutralizing antibody to MCP-1 inhibited the zymosan-induced increase in monocytes present in the peritoneum. Thus, MCP-1 is an important mediator of monocyte recruitment in this model of inflammation.

In addition to their potential pro-inflammatory actions, a presentation by B. Strum described the potential of novel chemokine to provide some modest protection in endotoxin model of shock. M-CIF or HCC-1 or MIP-1γ or CKβ-1 partially protected BALB/c mice against the lethality induced by the administration of 25 mg/kg but not 50 mg/kg of LPS. The mechanism for this protection may be the reduction in serum TNF seen after administration of this chemokine. These intriguing but preliminary findings need to be verified to further our understanding of the role of chemokines in the pathophysiology of inflammatory disease.

The final presentation of the evening by Dr. R.J. Collins discussed the role of MCP-1 in the recruitment of inflammatory cells in delayed type hypersensitivity reactions. Using a hamster anti-mouse MCP-1 antibody, Dr. Collins demonstrated a reduction in ear swelling and the cellular influx after DNFB challenge in sensitized mice. Furthermore, using an antagonist of MCP-1 binding to monocytes, SA067 (IC_{50} = .0 µM), Dr. Collins showed that administration of SA067 (50 mg/kg, i.p.) at the time of challenge and subsequently every 2 h for the next 12 h produced a substantial reduction in ear swelling. This exciting result represents the first demonstration that a receptor antagonist for the chemokine can inhibit an inflammatory condition and thus provides impetus to identify more potent and long lasting antagonists for these interesting families of proteins.

AAS 49
Therapeutic Strategies for Modulating the Inflammatory Diseases
© 1998 Birkhäuser Verlag Basel/Switzerland

Intracellular signaling processes

A. Kazlauskas (Harvard) and K. Hulkower (Abbott)

The talks presented in this workshop focused on various aspects of intracellular signal transduction and were a good complement to topics presented by speakers at the morning symposium on intracellular signaling. The workshop talks were organized into two major subject areas with the first four speakers examining signaling pathways involved in pro-inflammatory responses in several cellular and *in vivo* settings. Dr. K. Hulkower (Abbott Labs) described his studies in human amnionic WISH cells in which there appear to be different signal transduction pathways utilized by these cells to induce prostaglandin H synthase-2 (PGHS-2) depending upon the stimulus used to elicit PGE_2 production. These cells were also found to produce tumor necrosis factor-α (TNF-α) in addition to PGE_2, however this occurred through a completely different signal transduction pathway than that used by the cells for the induction of PGHS-2. Dr. M. Holly (Roche) used a system in which activation of the stress pathway *via* interleukin-1 (IL-1) or TNF-α results in activation of the JNK/SEK-1 cascade and leads to expression of the matrix metalloproteinases (MMPs) stromelysin and collagenase. Murine fibroblasts expressing dominant negative SEK-1 or with SEK-1 activity otherwise inhibited resulted in significant decreases in MMP transcription induced by IL-1 or TNF-α. Dr. P. Scherle (DuPont-Merck) demonstrated that IL-1 activates all three of the well characterized MAPK family members, ERK, JNK and p38, in rabbit articular chondrocytes and that maximal activation of ERK and p38 occurs at 1 ng/ml of IL-1. A ten-fold higher concentration of IL-1 was required to elicit maximal activation of JNK. Additional studies indicated that the MAPK family members could be selectively activated with phorbol dibutyrate and TNF while there was no effect in response to LPS and transforming growth factor-β (TGF-β). Using the classic *in vivo* model of TPA-induced ear edema in mice, Dr. E. Tancula (DuPont-Merck) showed that the TPA stimulated a delayed and prolonged activation of MEK/ERK in the ear homogenate which was tightly correlated with the swelling response. It was thought that the sustained nature of this response was due to the influx of neutrophils. Interestingly, indomethacin, a classic non-steroidal antiinflammatory drug (NSAID) which inhibits swelling in this model did not block the activation of ERK in the ear homogenate.

The second major subject area covered by the last three workshop speakers focused on the examination of signaling through specific cellular or cytokine receptors. Dr. J. Rediske (CIBA) challenged bovine articular chondrocytes with fibronectin-coated latex beads which bind to the fibronectin receptor, a5b1 integrin. This caused a clustering of the receptors and assembly of a complex consisting of F-actin, the focal adhesion kinase (FAK), the G-protein RhoA and tyrosine phosphorylated proteins. Exogenous NO or NO inducing cytokines such as IL-1 and TNF inhibited formation of this complex while not affecting total fibronectin bead binding or clustering of the receptor. The effects of the cytokines were reversed by an NO synthase inhibitor demonstrating a mechanism for the effect of NO on chondrocyte-matrix interactions. Dr. P. Changelian (Pfizer) described studies in which his group established an ELISA based screen for inhibitors of JAK3 tyrosine kinase signaling. The assay included the use of tyrosine containing peptides derived from subunits of the IL-2 receptor, IL-4 receptor, STAT6 and JAK1 as substrates, all of which are known to interact with the catalytic domain of JAK3. This screen has already produced a hit which inhibits IL-2 stimulated STAT 5 phosphorylation. Mr. J. Foley (SmithKline Beecham) described studies in which his group has cloned and characterized the human anaphylatoxin C3a receptor which previously was only known as a 7 transmembrane domain, G-protein coupled "orphan" receptor. The receptor was expressed in RBL-2H3 cells and found to have identical properties to the native C3a receptor found on human neutrophils. Inhibitor studies indicate that the C3a receptor couples to a pertussis-sensitive G protein and to phospholipase C.

Recent studies have demonstrated that intracellular signal transduction pathways which control inflammatory processes involve many members from distinct families of protein kinases. Consequently, these kinases represent achievable targets for therapeutic intervention. This workshop highlighted both the significant progress of pharmaceutical discovery programs, as well as the need to continue basic research in the area of intracellular signal relay that regulates inflammation.

AAS 49
Therapeutic Strategies for Modulating the Inflammatory Diseases
© 1998 Birkhäuser Verlag Basel/Switzerland

Immunology of inflammation

R. de Waal Malefyt (DNAX) and Z. Jonak (SmithKline Beecham)

Experimental allergic encephalomyelitis (EAE) models in drug discovery

EAE is a murine model of multiple sclerosis in which autoimmune tissue destruction and demyelination is mediated by myelin basic protein specific T-cells belonging to the T helper 1 subset and can develop from acute to chronic phases.

Dr. Anthony Milici (Pfizer) discussed his results on the role of eosinophils in the optic nerve of SJL mice with EAE. Disease was induced in these mice by i.p. injection of encephalogenic T-cells. The authors observed an influx of eosinophils in the optic nerve which resulted in a total of 22% non-neuronal tissue present during the the the acute phase of the disease. The eosinophil influx occurred on day 7 after transfer of T-cells and decreased to background levels by day 10. It is thought that products of eosinophils such as neurotoxin and cationic protein are responsible for some of the demyelinating effects. Eosinophil infiltration was also evident with the onset of flares.

The next two presentations described the use of new drugs which interfered with the development or showed activity in treating autoimmune disease models such as EAE (mouse and rat), Collagen Induced Arthritis (CIA) (DBA mice), and Adjuvant Arthritis (AA) (rats). PNU 156804 is a synthetic Prodigiosin derivative with reduced toxicity and tested for immunosuppressive activity by Drs. Ferrari and Fornasiero (Pharmacia & Upjohn). *In vitro*, PNU 156804 specifically inhibited the proliferation of T-cells to IL-2, IL-4, IL-7 and IL-15, but not to GM-CSF and IL-3. In addition, PNU 156804 inhibited activities of the former cytokines on B-cells. *In vivo*, this compound blocked the onset of EAE in mice and rats. PNU 156804 reduced the acute phase of EAE and prevented relapses. In contrast, animals treated with CsA did relapse after withdrawal. AA was significantly reduced by PNU 156804 and low doses of PNU 156804 and CsA acted synergistically to inhibit disease. Finally, PNU 156804 increased graft survival of heart allo-transplants in the rat for over 35 days. One potential mechanism of PNU 156804 may be interference of interactions between the common g chain and IL-2/IL-4/IL-7/IL-9 receptor or its association/activation with JAK3 kinase.

Dr. Schörlemmer (Behringwerke) discussed the activities of MNA 279 and MNA 715, derivatives of the leflunomide metabolite A771726 in acute and chronic models of relapsing EAE in rats and in Biozzi (outbred) mice. Both MNA 279 and MNA 715 did not prevent the development of disease but delayed the onset and reduced the symptoms of acute EAE in rats. In relapsing models of EAE in rats and mice, both compounds delayed the onset of the first episode and prevented relapse to second and third episodes. These drugs could also be used in therapeutic treatments if they were administered after the first episode. The compounds could be administered orally and appeared to act in a dose dependent manner. *In vitro*, these compounds inhibited T- and B-cell proliferation and Ab production. Both drugs were also immunosuppressive in SLE and graft *versus* host disease. However, the exact mechanism of action for these drugs is not known.

Cytokines in autoimmune diseases

The group of Wim van der Berg (Univ. Hospital Nijmegen) discussed the role of IL-4, IL-10 and IL-12 in an acute (SCW in C57Bl) and a chronic (collagen type II in DBA-1) model of Arthritis. In the acute model, IL-10 reduced joint swelling, TNF and IL-1β synthesis and enhanced chondrocyte derived PG synthesis whereas IL-4 by itself was not active. However combinations of IL-10 and IL-4 were synergistic in reduction of joint swelling, TNF, and IL-1 synthesis. Administration of anti-IL-4 mAbs prior to challenge did not affect the response to SCW, but anti-IL-10 mAbs or anti-IL-10 and anti-IL-4 mAbs enhanced joint swelling and strongly inhibited PG synthesis, indicating that the response is regulated by endogenously produced IL-10. A similar synergy between IL-4 and IL-10 in reducing Th1 responses was also demonstrated in a model of Leishmania major infection by Fiona Powrie and Bob Coffman at DNAX. In a Th1 mediated chronic model of arthritis a similar synergy in reducing the response between IL-4 and IL-10 was observed following rechallenge of the animals at day 28. IL-10 alone also inhibited this response partially. The course of arthritis can be accelerated by administration of IL-1, TNF, TGFb or LPS at day 28 and this acceleration could be inhibited by antibodies to IL-12. Conversely, IL-12 could also accelerate the response. Interestingly, later addition (day 35) of IL-12 led to an amelioration of the response whereas addition of anti-IL-12 antibodies led to an acceleration of the response. This correlated with an increase and a decrease of IL-10 levels respectively and the acceleration of the response with anti-IL-12 mAbs could be reversed by administration of IL-10 indicating that in later phases of this chronic response a balance between IL-12 and IL-10 (Th1/Th2) still exists and can be modulated. The induction of IL-10 by IL-12 has also recently been reported in *in vitro* experiments with human T-cells.

   Dr. Williams (Univ. of Pennsylvania) showed that CDR1 peptides derived from GM-CSF inhibited the binding of GM-CSF to its receptor. These peptides were derived *via* determination of contact residues between GM-CSF and its receptor or based on a light chain mimic of GM-CSF. GM-CSF upregulates HLA-DR expression in rheumatoid arthritis and these peptides could be a way to intervene with the inflammatory process in the joint. Using synovial cells as APC, several T-cell lines were established from RA patients. These T-cell lines had selective expansion of Vβ12 and Vβ5 or Vβ8 for a CD8 positive line. These lines reacted with antigens present in crude cartilage extracts and may play an important role as autoreactive cells in the inflammation. These lines may be useful in determining the auto-antigen in RA. No information was available on the cytokine production of these cells.

Use of humanized mAbs

Dr. Simon Blake (Celltech Therapeutics) reported on his studies with a humanized anti-E selectin mAb that prevents leukocyte rolling on activated endothelium and thus subsequent extravasation of neutrophils in the tissues. The antibody did not induce ADCC or complement lysis due to its engineering to the IgG4 subclass which does not interact with FcR. The antibody inhibited infiltration of human skin transplanted in SCID mice and in baboons following TNF injection. Pharmacokinetics indicated a half-life of 12–14 days and no evidence was found for the production of auto antibodies.

AAS 49
Therapeutic Strategies for Modulating the Inflammatory Diseases
© 1998 Birkhäuser Verlag Basel/Switzerland

Lipid and peptide mediators and their enzymes

S.G. Farmer (Zeneca)

Three presentations dealt with transgenic modification of enzymes involved in eicosanoid biosynthesis. David Grass (DNX Transgenics) described mice (B6xDBA1 and C57BL/65) made transgenic (*tg*) for human Group II phospholipase A_2 (GpIIPLA$_2$). Wild types do not express detectable GpIIPLA$_2$. GpIIPLA$_2$-*tg* mice are characterized by severe hyperkeratosis, alopecia and epidermal hyperplasia although no inflammatory cells were found in skin, and animals exhibited no increase in "spontaneous" arthritis. GpIIPLA$_2$-*tg* mice were highly sensitive to endotoxin-induced death, albeit the underlying mechanisms (shock, leukocyte-mediated organ damage) are unknown. Effects of drugs were not examined in *tg* mice, although drugs that interfere with prostaglandins (PG), leukotrienes (LT) or platelet-activating factor (PAF) are beneficial in other models of endotoxin shock. GpIIPLA$_2$-*tg* mice were bred with a strain expressing human tumor necrosis factor-α (TNF). The double-*tg* progeny exhibit increased susceptibility to joint distortion and paw edema. Furthermore, arthritis has earlier onset and greater severity than in single TNF-*tg* mice. Thus, GpIIPLA$_2$-*tg* animals have increased sensitivity to induced arthritis. Serum HDL-cholesterol is reduced in chronic inflammation, and evidence suggests that GpIIPLA$_2$-*tg* is involved in lipoprotein metabolism and initiation of atherosclerosis. GpIIPLA$_2$-*tg* mice exhibit 25–40% decreases in serum HDL compared with wild types, but no change in LDL. When fed a high-fat diet for 18 weeks, female *tg* mice manifested around a four-fold greater incidence of atherosclerotic lesions than controls. These mice will prove useful in testing novel PLA$_2$ inhibitors, and to study the role of GpIIPLA$_2$-*tg* in inflammatory and vascular diseases. Further characterization of this strain, e.g., with cyclooxygenase and lipoxygenase inhibitors, is anticipated. Dr. Grass noted, however, that GpIIPLA$_2$-*tg* mice make "lousy mothers" and breeding may not yield optimal litter sizes or survival.

Two presentations examined *tg*-knockout (*ko*), respectively, of cyclooxygenase-2 (COX-2) and 5-lipoxygenase-activating protein (FLAP), with notably contrasting effects on the health of mice. Whereas COX-1 is expressed constitutively in all tissues, and has important roles in homeostasis, COX-2 is induced in leukocytes and may be involved in inflammation and host defense. COX-2 is thought to be responsible for PG production in inflammation. Jim Trzaskos (DuPont Merck) described *ko* mice following targeted disruption of the COX-2 gene. COX-2-*ko* mice have impaired fertility and development, with markedly reduced litters, and developmental renal dysplasia and myocardial fibrosis. PGs are required for normal ovulation, implantation and parturition, and nonselective inhibitors of COX-1/2, like indomethacin, impair fertility. Trzaskos et al. demonstrated that COX-2-*ko* mice exhibit abnormal decidualization and a low rate of implantation. This probably causes infertility. Conversely, PMA- and carrageenan-induced edema, PG-driven models of inflammation, are normal in COX-2-*ko* mice (*Nature*, 378: 4006-409, 1995). Thus, COX-2 is necessary for maternal PG production and establishment of pregnancy, but its role in inflammation (at least in mice) may not be as critical.

Richard Griffiths (Pfizer) and co-workers created an embryonic stem cell line from DBA1 mice that permits deletion of the FLAP gene in a strain of mouse that is susceptible to collagen-induced arthritis (CIA). FLAP is required for activation of 5-LO and LT biosynthesis. No phenotype abnormalities were evident in FLAP-*ko* mice and, unlike COX-2-*ko* mice, FLAP deficient animals exhibit normal fertility and development. Injection of zymosan i.p. generates local eicosanoids and plasma extravasation in normal mice. In contrast, although FLAP-*ko* mice exhibit a normal PG response to zymosan, LT biosynthesis is abolished and extravasation reduced by 50–60%. He noted that there is a similar reduction of zymosan peritonitis in 5-LO-*ko* and FLAP-*ko* animals. Also, like GpIIPLA$_2$-*tg* mice, FLAP- and 5-LO-depleted mice are more susceptible to endotoxin lethality, indicating important roles for LTs in this model of sepsis. Furthermore, the severity of CIA in FLAP-*ko* animals was reduced by over 70%. These results convincingly indicate that products of 5-LO are pivotal in the development of CIA in mice. Unlike the case with COX-2-*ko*, however, where PGs are necessary for normal development and homeostasis, LTs do not seem to be singularly important in those regards, but are required for initiation and maintenance of inflammation.

Jeff Jackson and colleagues (SmithKline Beecham) examined effects of drugs on angiogenesis of adjuvant-induced granulomas in rat skin air pouches. Inhibition of GpIIPLA$_2$ reduced angiogenesis without altering granuloma weight, whereas 5-LO inhibition reduced granuloma growth but had no effect on angiogenesis. Thus, while LTs may play a role in granuloma formation, other arachidonate metabolites may be more important in neovascularization. It will be interesting to determine whether angiogenesis is altered in *tg* mice deficient in 5-LO or GpIIPLA. Medroxyprogesterone, an angiostatic drug, and protamine, which binds heparin, both reduced angiogenesis without affecting granuloma growth. The ability of these agents to reduce TNF and IL-1 production was noted as a possible mechanism underlying their angiostasis. Jackson also reported that batimistat, a matrix metalloprotease inhibitor, stimulated angiogenesis while reducing granuloma development.

Thivierge and colleagues (University of Sherbrooke) examined differential regulation by interferon-γ (IFN), a Th1 cytokine, and IL-4 and IL-10, Th2 cytokines, on expression of monocyte receptors for lipid and peptide mediators of chemotaxis. PMA inhibited PAF receptor expression *via* protein kinase C, and augmented receptor mRNA degradation. In contrast, PMA increased C5a receptor expression. IFN inhibited C5a receptor expression, and increased PAF and fMLP receptor expression. Similarly, IL-10 inhibited expression of C5a receptors, augmented fMLP receptor expression, but was without effect on PAF receptors. IL-4 decreased both gene and protein expression for C5a receptors whereas the cytokine increased expression of receptors for PAF but, curiously, decreased PAF receptor mRNA.

Three presentations involved the inflammatory peptide, bradykinin (BK). Stephen Farmer and associates (Zeneca) describe for the first time the cloning and functional expression of a guinea pig BK lung receptor which shares >80% sequence homology with human, rat and mouse B_2 receptors. Its C-terminus has an extra 8 amino acids not present in other species. cDNA was expressed in CHO-K1 cells, and binding studies indicate that the cloned receptor is a B_2 subtype. In CHO cells expressing the guinea pig receptor all ligands, including several known antagonists, were full or partial agonists of $^{45}Ca^{2+}$ efflux, possibly due to over-expression. The authors noted that the existence of the putative guinea pig B_2 receptor remains controversial.

Pierre Farmer (Sherbrooke) studied kinin receptor subtypes mediating increased permeability of bovine aortic endothelial cells (BAEC). BK-induced albumin clearance is inhibited by a B_2 antagonist. In addition, specific B_1 receptor agonists were without effect, indicating that BK-induced hyperpermeability is mediated *via* B_2 receptors. Following 24 h preincubation with IL-1, which has been shown in other cell types to upregulate B_1 receptor expression, BAEC responded to B_1 agonists, whereas responses to BK itself were unaffected. Finally, Pasternak and colleagues (New Jersey Medical School) examined blood coagulation in the presence of 50 nM BK. Blood containing BK for 10 or 120 min coagulated at the same rate as control blood whereas, in the presence of endotoxin, clotting time was reduced from 5.8 to 5 min. It was suggested that BK may interact with endotoxin-stimulated monocytes to release tissue factor. In Gram-negative sepsis, the kinin and coagulation systems are activated, and there may be microthrombus formation. However, kinins are degraded very rapidly (<1 min) to pharmacologically inactive fragments in blood, and whether this procoagulant effect is receptor-mediated or even specific is doubtful.

Subject Index

acute graft versus host disease (aGVHD) 20
adjuvant arthritis 91
airway 67
airway hyperreactivity 70
anti-CD3 37
anti-CD40 17
anti-CD28 mAb 37
anti-CTLA-4 mAb 37
anti-IFNγ antibody 62
anti-IL-4 mAb 102
anti-IL-10 mAb 102
anti-TNF antibody 87, 88
anti-TNFα 62
antigen presenting cells (APCs) 23
antigen receptor (TCR) 23
antigen-specific T-cell tolerance 23
AP-1 83
apoptosis 2
arthritis, rat adjuvant 46
autoimmune disease 40

B lymphocyte 10
B-cell 18
B7-1 15
B7-2 15
B7-CD28/CTLA-4 pathway 40

C3a receptor 100
C5a 3, 107
C5aR deficient mice 3
carrageenan induced paw edema 46
cartilage protection agent (CPA) 45, 49
Caspase-1 1
Caspase-2 1
CCR1 95
CCR3 95
CCR5 3, 95
CD3/TCR signaling 33
CD4$^+$ T cell 9, 17
CD8$^+$ T cell 9, 34, 59
CD20 17
CD28 15, 24
CD28 deficient mice 24, 35
CD40 15, 24
CD40 deficient mice 18
CD80 58
CD86 58
celecoxib (SC-58635) 46
chemokine 60, 95

colitis 46
corticosteroid, inhaled 75
CPP32 2
Crohn's disease 46, 57
CTLA-4 15, 16, 33
CTLA-4 deficient mice 15, 37
cyclooxygenase (COX) 77
    COX-1 46, 77
    COX-2 46, 77
    COX-2 inhibitor 46, 92
cytokine synthesis inhibition factor (CSIF) 57

D-NAME 75
hypersensitivity, delayed type 61
delayed-type hypersensitivity reaction (DTHR)
   25, 61
diphosphonate (DP) 80
disease modifying anti-rheumatic drug
   (DMARD) 49

eosinophil 70
Epstein Barr virus 57
experimental autoimmune encephalomyelitis
   (EAE) model 3

fas 38
fibroblast 10
fibronectin (FN) 81
focal adhesion kinase (FAK) 100

gelatinase A 45
gene expression 39
glucocorticoid hormone 84
glucocorticoid receptor (GR) 84
GM-CSF 101, 102
gp39 15, 18
GpIIPLA$_2$-*tg* 105
Gro-α 95
group II phospholipase A$_2$ (GpIIPLA$_2$) 105
growth factor 39

HIV-1 96
HLA-DR 103
horseradish peroxidase (HRP) 91
human leukocyte elastase (HLE) 92
Hyper-IgM syndrome (HIM) 17
hypoxia inducible factor-1 (HIF-1) 85

ICAM 46, 58
ICE deficient animal 8
IFN-γ 8, 26, 29
IgE 24

Progress in Inflammation Research

Series Editor: Michael J. Parnham

The Continuation of the Book Series
AGENTS and ACTIONS SUPPLEMENTS!

The last few years have seen a revolution in our understanding of how blood and tissue cells interact and of the intracellular mechanisms controlling their activation. This has not only provided multiple targets for potential anti-inflammatory and immuno-modulatory therapy, but has also revealed the underlying inflammatory pathology of many diseases.

This monograph series provides up-to-date information on the latest developments in the pathology, mechanisms and therapy of inflammatory disease. Areas covered include: vascular responses, skin inflammation, pain, neuroinflammation, arthritis cartilage and bone, airways inflammation and asthma, allergy, cytokines and inflammatory mediators, cell signalling, and recent advances in drug therapy. Each volume is edited by acknowledged experts providing succinct overviews on specific topics intended to inform and explain. The series is of interest to academic and industrial biomedical researchers, drug development personnel and rheumatologists, allergologists, pathologists, dermatologists and other clinicians requiring regular scientific updates.

Forthcoming titles:

Chemokines and skin
edited by E. Kownatzki and J. Norgauer
Cellular mechanisms in airways inflammation
edited by C. Page, K. Banner and D. Spina
Immunomodulatory agents from plants
edited by H. Wagner
Inducible enzymes in the inflammatory response
edited by D.A. Willoughby and A. Tomlinson
Gene Therapy in inflammatory diseases
edited by C.H. Evans and P. Robbins

For detailed information please see
http://www.birkhauser.ch
or mail to
sales@birkhauser.ch

Birkhäuser Verlag • Basel • Boston • Berlin

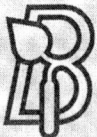